NUTS

AND

SEEDS

For my granddaughter, Elsie, who loves walnuts.

NUTS
AND
SEEDS

Improving Your Health

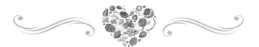

Patsy Westcott

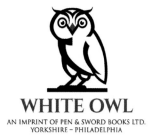

WHITE OWL
AN IMPRINT OF PEN & SWORD BOOKS LTD.
YORKSHIRE – PHILADELPHIA

First published in Great Britain in 2019 by
Pen and Sword WHITE OWL
An imprint of
Pen & Sword Books Ltd
Yorkshire - Philadelphia

ISBN 978 1 52672 588 2

A CIP catalogue record for this book is available from the British Library.

Typeset in 11/14 pts Palatino
by Aura Technology and Software Services, India

Printed and bound in India by Replika Press Pvt. Ltd.

Pen & Sword Books Ltd incorporates the Imprints of Pen & Sword Books Archaeology,
Atlas, Aviation, Battleground, Discovery, Family History, History, Maritime, Military,
Naval, Politics, Railways, Select, Transport, True Crime, Fiction, Frontline Books, Leo
Cooper, Praetorian Press, Seaforth Publishing, Wharncliffe and White Owl.

For a complete list of Pen & Sword titles please contact

PEN & SWORD BOOKS LIMITED
47 Church Street, Barnsley, South Yorkshire, S70 2AS, England
E-mail: enquiries@pen-and-sword.co.uk
Website: www.pen-and-sword.co.uk

or

PEN AND SWORD BOOKS
1950 Lawrence Rd, Havertown, PA 19083, USA
E-mail: Uspen-and-sword@casematepublishers.com
Website: www.penandswordbooks.com

Contents

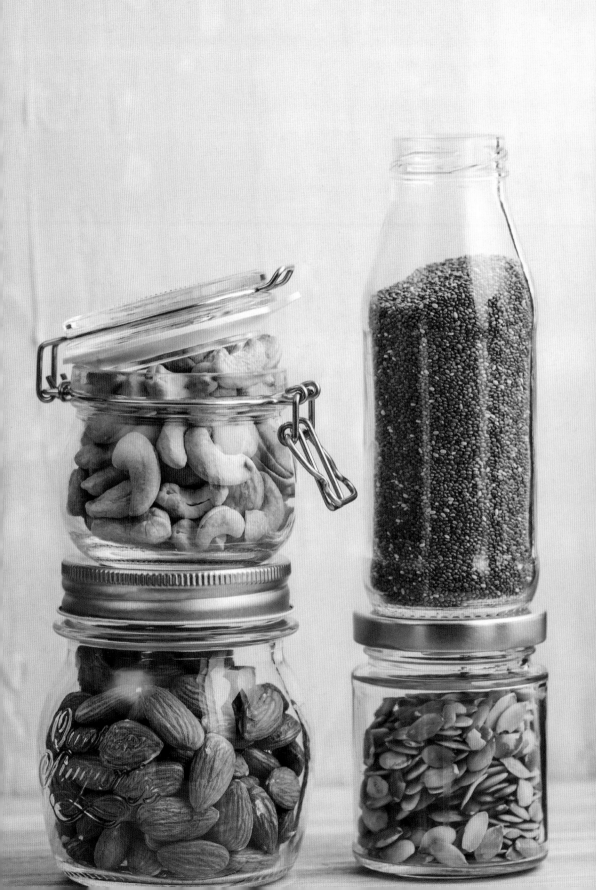

FOREWORD

Pick up any newspaper, switch on the TV, click on your Twitter or other social media feed and what do you see? Chances are, an item blazoning the health benefits of some food, diet or nutrient. But dig a bit deeper and you'll often discover there isn't a great deal of genuine scientific evidence to support the benefits claimed.

As someone with a passion for food – and a higher degree in nutritional medicine – I've little truck with headlines that hail a food as 'good' one week and dismiss that same food as 'bad' the next. Fortunately, when it comes to nuts and seeds, the story is pretty compelling. There is loads of evidence, for example, showing the wide-ranging benefits nuts can have for health. And it is becoming ever more apparent that nuts – and seeds – are bursting with exactly the right combination of nutrients we need to keep our bodies working as they should to help us stay healthy throughout life.

Of course, some of the studies out there are still at an early stage or show associations that can't be proved. That's why, in the pages that follow, I've tried to give you some idea of just where the research is at. To this end I've combed the science journals to find the strongest and most recent studies. And where a study has only been carried out in the test tube, in animals, or in a handful of people I've said so. That way I hope you'll be able to decide for yourself how much credence to give to what you read in the headlines. So here it is: your straight-talking guide to nuts and seeds. Let's get cracking.

ABOUT NUTS AND SEEDS

The importance of nuts and seeds as part of an optimum diet for our health and that of the planet can't be underestimated. Indeed, we humans have enjoyed snacking on them for millennia, as an exciting find at Israel's Gesher Benot Ya'aqov archaeology site in the eastern Mediterranean revealed back in 2002. There, archaeologists uncovered the remains of nuts, seeds, fruit, vegetables and tuberous roots together with the well-worn hammers and anvils used to crack open nutshells dating back some 780,000 years.

Evidently our Stone Age ancestors enjoyed something like the plant-based Mediterranean diet we're advised to eat for health today. Fast forward to the twenty-first century and we still can't get enough of nuts and seeds. Each of us chomps our way through almost 2 kilos a year. Even astronauts on missions apparently can't wait to get their hands on the peanut pouches (not strictly nuts though included as such) regularly shuttled out from the Space Station.

It's not hard to see why. Portable, compact, tasty and brimming with nutrients, many of whose benefits are still only now being uncovered, nuts and seeds, pack a super-healthy punch. No surprise then that they feature on some of the world's most fêted 'food pyramids', including America's Harvard Nutrition's Healthy Eating Pyramid, and the Mediterranean Diet Pyramid, which reflects what is consistently considered the healthiest eating pattern in the world.

But what exactly are nuts and seeds and what accounts for their potential health benefits? Simple question, right? But the answer turns out to be somewhat complicated. For a start, it depends who you ask. What's more, while most nuts are seeds, not all seeds are nuts. You'll be relieved to know then, that to keep things simple I've stuck with those you can easily find in the nuts and seeds section of the supermarket or health store. And, because I'm keen to bring you the latest science, this has the added advantage of them being the ones backed by the most solid evidence.

GROWING EVIDENCE

The good news is: there's now a huge and growing body of evidence to suggest that people who consume a diet containing nuts and, to a lesser extent seeds (simply

HEALTHY EATING PYRAMID

Department of Nutrition, Harvard School of Public Health

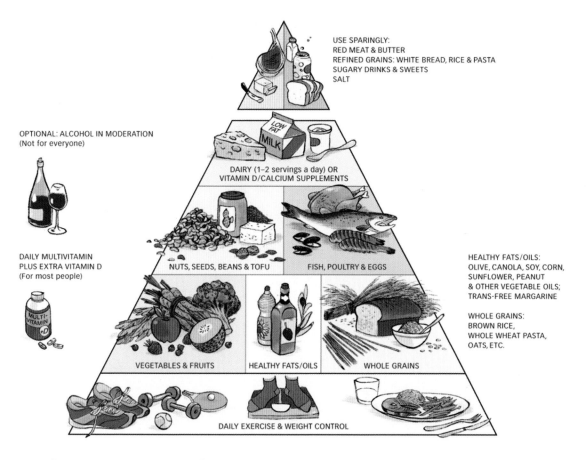

USE SPARINGLY:
RED MEAT & BUTTER
REFINED GRAINS: WHITE BREAD, RICE & PASTA
SUGARY DRINKS & SWEETS
SALT

OPTIONAL: ALCOHOL IN MODERATION
(Not for everyone)

DAIRY (1–2 servings a day) OR
VITAMIN D/CALCIUM SUPPLEMENTS

DAILY MULTIVITAMIN
PLUS EXTRA VITAMIN D
(For most people)

NUTS, SEEDS, BEANS & TOFU

FISH, POULTRY & EGGS

HEALTHY FATS/OILS:
OLIVE, CANOLA, SOY, CORN,
SUNFLOWER, PEANUT
& OTHER VEGETABLE OILS;
TRANS-FREE MARGARINE

WHOLE GRAINS:
BROWN RICE,
WHOLE WHEAT PASTA,
OATS, ETC.

VEGETABLES & FRUITS

HEALTHY FATS/OILS

WHOLE GRAINS

DAILY EXERCISE & WEIGHT CONTROL

because we consume less of them) have better health and live longer. A large overview of studies, by researchers from London's Imperial College, for example, found that that just 20 grams of nuts a day – equivalent to a handful – can cut the risk of coronary heart disease by nearly 30 per cent, of cancer by 15 per cent, and of dying early by 22 per cent. An average of at least this same amount of nuts was also linked with an approximately 50 per cent lower risk of dying from respiratory disease, and almost 40 per cent lower risk of dying of diabetes, although as they admit, there is less information about these diseases.

What's interesting about this is that these are all examples of the so-called non-communicable diseases (NCDs) the World Health Organisation has earmarked to reduce deaths from by a third by 2030. And there is also emerging research that

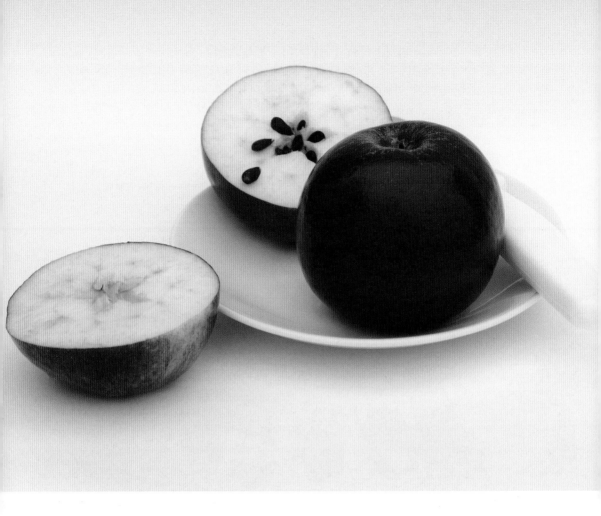

nuts and seeds can help protect against neurodegenerative diseases, which affect the brain and nervous system, such as Alzheimer's disease, vascular dementia and Parkinson's disease. Indeed, according to a review published in the journal *Food and Function,* they may help to slow down - and even, although this seems a taller order, reverse - the ageing process.

These are big claims, but they make sense when you consider that many such diseases often have common origins in terms of what's going on inside our bodies. Oxidation, sometimes called oxidative stress, the same process that turns butter rancid, an apple brown when you cut it and leave it open to the air, or iron rusty - the human equivalent of rusting if you like - is one such process.

But that's not all. In recent years another key player has emerged as a potentially powerful driver of disease and ageing: inflammation. Inflammation is not a bad thing in itself, it's a normal response to injury. But if it continues unchecked month after month, year after year, it can damage cells and lead to disease. As a source of

NUTS AND SEEDS

antioxidant and anti-inflammatory nutrients, nuts and seeds may exert a modifying influence on both these processes, one possible explanation for why they consistently come out tops in studies.

A WEIGHTY ISSUE

Before digging deeper, let's get one thing straight. Not so long ago advice on nuts was invariably accompanied by a sentence along the lines of 'Don't overdo them as they are high in fat and calories which can pile on the pounds.' And it's true that they are highly calorific – from around 550 kcals per 100 grams in almonds, cashews and pistachios, to more than 700 kcals per 100 grams in macadamias.

However, the quality of nutrients you get for those calories is unbeatable. Nuts are a compact store of all the nutrients needed to grow a new plant or tree. As such they are a rich source of all three of the large groups of nutrients – what nutritional scientists call macronutrients – that is carbohydrates, protein and fat – as well as a host of micronutrients, that is vitamins and minerals, plus plant or phytonutrients including many different types of fibre-needed to support health and fend off disease.

In fact, returning to that line about them piling on the pounds, studies now suggest that, not only does this not stand up to scrutiny, but that they may actually help *lower* the risk of weight gain. How so? It is still not known exactly, but one theory is that, as a rich source of fat and protein, they help increase that nice, satisfied feeling of having had enough to eat we get after meals – what the experts call satiety. Another is that because they contain fibre which passes undigested to our colon, not all the calories in nuts are absorbed. Whatever the reason, according to two of the most respected US researchers to examine the matter it seems that replacing unhealthy snacks, such as biscuits, cakes, crisps and so on, with a daily handful of nuts to keep weight in check could be a smart move.

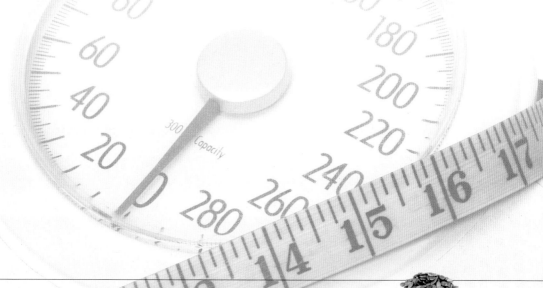

A NUTRITIONAL DETECTIVE STORY

The story of how nuts came to be recognised as having such potentially powerful health benefits reads like a nutritional whodunnit. It began in earnest in the mid-twentieth century, when scientists in the US set out to investigate the health and lifestyle of members of the Church of the Seventh Day Adventists, a group of people famed for their longevity and freedom from common lifestyle diseases. Most Adventists don't smoke or drink alcohol and many eat a mainly vegetarian diet. The scientists wanted to know: could their diet be part of their secret?

In the 1960s the US, in common with most of the Western world, was gripped by a seemingly unstoppable epidemic of heart disease. One of the first things the researchers did was look at the influence of the Adventist diet on cardiovascular problems, and by 1992 they had some exciting findings. Among 31,208 Californian

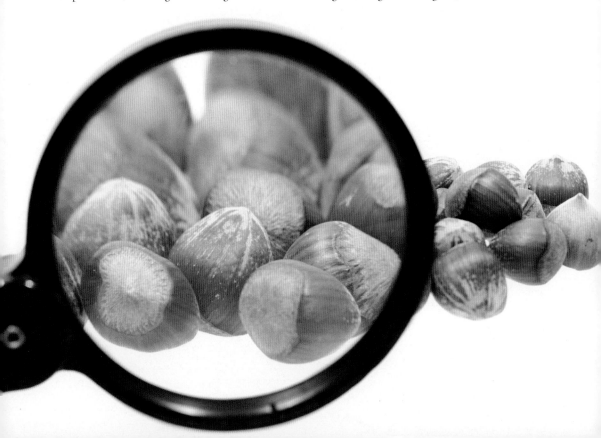

Adventists studied, those who ate nuts one to four times a week had a 26 per cent lower risk of having a heart attack and a 27 per cent lower risk of dying from heart disease compared with those who ate nuts less than once a week.

Those who ate nuts five or more times a week, meanwhile, had almost half the risk of a heart attack (a 48 per cent reduction in risk) and were more than a quarter (27 per cent) less likely to die, compared to those who consumed nuts less than once a week. A pretty impressive result. Nuts appeared to protect both vegetarians and non-vegetarians, although meat eaters seemed to benefit less.

Subsequent results from the Adventist study have included the finding that over the course of a lifetime, men who consume nuts five times a week or more have a 12 per cent lower risk of heart disease. And, even those who do eventually develop heart problems, appear to delay their onset by five or six years if they eat nuts frequently. It's not often a study can be described as genuinely groundbreaking, but this one was – and is; a second Adventist study (AHS-2) is producing findings to this day. Over the years it has allowed researchers to ask and answer searching questions as to how diet and lifestyle affect our health.

Numerous other studies now support the observations made by the Adventist researchers, including three famous large, long-running studies, the Nurses' Health Study (1980-2012), which included 76,364 women, the Nurses' Health Study II (1991-2013), which included 92,946 women, and the Health Professionals Follow-Up Study (1986-2012), which included 41,526 men. All these show strong links between nut consumption and a lower risk of heart disease. In fact, so convincing are the findings of these and other studies that the US Food and Drug Administration (FDA), a body not exactly known for wild pronouncements, has endorsed nuts in a health claim that states eating a small amount (specifically 1.5 oz or 43 grams) of most nuts a day as part of a diet low in saturated fat and cholesterol may reduce the risk of heart disease.

MEDITERRANEAN MAGIC

Fast forward to the twenty-first century and there is more compelling evidence for the benefits of nuts, this time from a large Spanish prevention trial which set out to examine the effects of two Mediterranean-style diets. One diet had added extra-virgin olive oil (around a litre a week), the other included 30 grams a day of added mixed nuts. These were compared to a low-fat diet recommended to reduce cardiovascular disease risk when the trial was first conceived in 2003.

In case you're interested the nuts in question were 15 grams of walnuts, 7.5 grams of hazelnuts and 7.5 grams almonds and the participants were 7,477 men and women aged 55-75 years and 60-80 years respectively. Although free of heart disease at the start of the study, they were all considered to have a high risk of developing it.

Originally set to last for six years, the study – called PREDIMED – Spanish for PREvención con DIeta MEDiterránea – was called to a halt just shy of the five-year

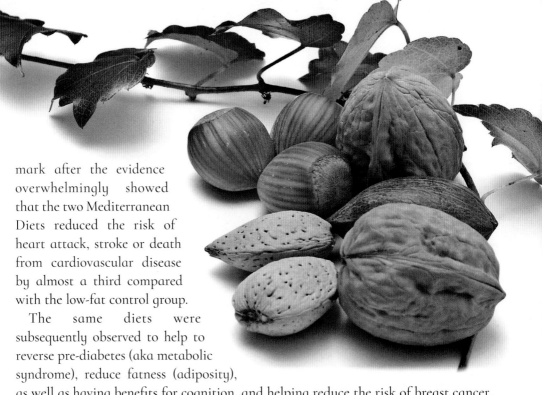

mark after the evidence overwhelmingly showed that the two Mediterranean Diets reduced the risk of heart attack, stroke or death from cardiovascular disease by almost a third compared with the low-fat control group.

The same diets were subsequently observed to help to reverse pre-diabetes (aka metabolic syndrome), reduce fatness (adiposity), as well as having benefits for cognition, and helping reduce the risk of breast cancer, and type 2 diabetes and its complications. The Mediterranean Diet with added nuts, meanwhile, also halved the risk of peripheral arterial disease (PAD), thickening and narrowing of the arteries serving the legs and arms, and of, atrial fibrillation, an especially dangerous arrhythmia or irregular heartbeat, which can cause blood clots and lead to a higher risk of stroke, and of heart failure, when the heart no longer has the strength to pump blood around the body.

One of the many revolutionary things about the PREDIMED trial is that it was one of the first large scale studies to focus on an overall dietary pattern – that is all the foods we eat, rather than single foods or nutrients. Nutritionists these days consider this to be much more accurate and reflective of the way we eat in the real world as well as a lesson in how to eat to maximise the synergy between different nutrients.

As persuasive – and headline grabbing – as these studies are, they are all what's known as 'observational', meaning that researchers trawl through the data of large groups of people to try and pinpoint links between the foods they eat and what happens to their health. Although they can identify such links or associations, however, what they can't do is tell us that a particular food (in this case nuts) *causes* a particular outcome (in this case a lower risk of heart disease).

To try and decide this, nutrition scientists need to do other types of studies and take these into account as part of a whole body of evidence. In the individual entries that follow you'll discover how some of these are contributing to what we know about nuts and seeds.

THE SECRET OF NUTS AND SEEDS

What makes nuts and seeds so healthy? Well, for a start, thanks to a plentiful supply of nutrients all working together or in synergy, they are what experts call 'complete functional foods' - that is 'foods that deliver additional or enhanced benefits over and above their basic nutritional value', if you want the official definition.

Nutritionally speaking, nuts and seeds contain similar nutrients. These are designed to protect their cells' genetic material or DNA, and ensure the plant or tree grows and develops into a strong, healthy specimen. Just like human beings, each type of nut or seed has a slightly different profile. So, while you may have your favourites, it's a good idea to include a wide variety of different ones in your diet to ensure you benefit from the various nutrients they contain and the synergy between them.

To pin this down a bit more precisely, nuts and seeds contain all three of the main nutrient groups - that is carbohydrates, fat and protein - in optimal amounts for health. Experts call these macronutrients - macro is Greek for large - because they are nutrients we need in large quantities.

Most nuts and seeds are relatively low in carbohydrates, but relatively high in fats, especially the monounsaturated fatty acids (MUFAs) and polyunsaturated fatty acids (PUFAs) linked to a lower risk of heart disease. Indeed, much of the research on nuts and seeds has, until fairly recently, focused mainly on their fatty acid content in relation to heart health, although this is beginning to change as scientists discover more about the benefits of other nutrients they contain. You can find out more in the individual entries and on pages 122 and 123.

Nuts and seeds are also rich in protein and amino acids, the building blocks of protein, needed to maintain and repair our cells, tissues and organs. And, intriguingly, while a high protein intake from red and processed meat seems to increase our risk of disease, the plant proteins found in nuts appear to lower it. It's not known exactly why, but it's thought that the levels and ratio of certain amino acids in nuts compared with that in animal sources of protein could have benefits especially in protecting against the oxidative stress and inflammation thought to play a role in many chronic diseases.

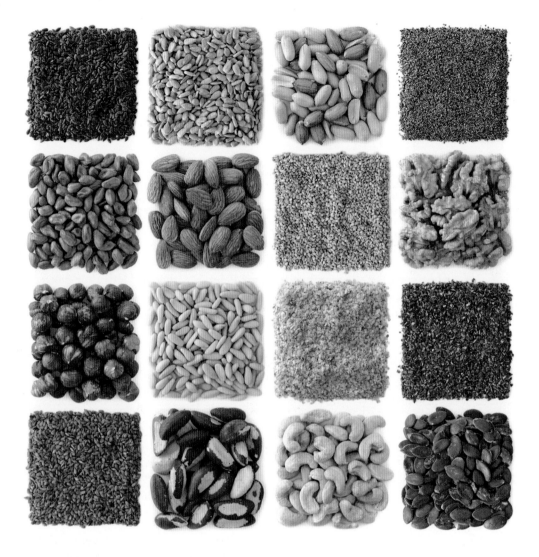

MICRONUTRIENTS AND MORE

Nuts and seeds are also a good source of micronutrients, vitamins and minerals such as vitamins A and C that together with vitamin E are part of the traditional triumvirate of antioxidant vitamins. Other micronutrients abundant in nuts include vitamin K, folate, and the B vitamin, thiamine, as well as minerals, such as calcium, iron, magnesium, phosphorus, potassium, zinc, and trace elements, such as copper and selenium.

In recent years nutritional scientists have begun increasingly to turn their attention to the arsenal of biologically active plant compounds – or phytonutrients – nuts and seeds contain, especially a huge class of these called polyphenols. These are produced by plants to defend themselves against threats from parasites, pests and disease, whose benefits we humans essentially hijack when we eat foods of plant origin. Indeed, polyphenols are widely linked with a lower risk of several degenerative diseases, including heart disease, type 2 diabetes, osteoporosis, degenerative diseases affecting the brain and nervous system and cancers, although there's a lot of research still to be done to work out exactly how they may confer their benefits.

But what accounts for these effects? Until fairly recently most scientists thought it was down to their antioxidant properties. But one thing was puzzling. Polyphenols break down pretty quickly in our bodies and are poorly absorbed and processed extremely fast, meaning that they are not easily taken up and used or bioavailable. There must be some other way in which they exert their apparent benefits.

In recent years the spotlight has increasingly turned on the chemical by-products – what scientists call secondary metabolites - produced by polyphenols. These can be produced in the course of a plant's normal development, in response to stress, or processing either in the food factory or the kitchen. For example, researchers writing in *Food Chemistry* reported that the antioxidant potential was greatest in Brazil nuts when raw, pistachios when toasted and in cashews when fried. So variety on the way you consume nuts is as important as variety in types of nuts.

And that's not all. Some of the most important of these secondary compounds are produced right there in our bodies. Indeed, there's increasing evidence to suggest that health benefits linked to polyphenols depend to a large extent on their transformation by our own gut bacteria into these chemicals. Researchers are now trying to tease out exactly how these may act by triggering the body's own internal antioxidant systems or helping keep a lid on inflammation, for example.

Now you can't move these days in the nutritional world without bumping into the gut microbiome – the sum total of bacteria, fungi and other minute organisms that inhabit our large intestine or colon – and its important role in health and disease. And here too it seems that nuts and seeds are right on the money. The reason? In a word: fibre, a much neglected nutrient in recent years.

In 2019 a new study commissioned by the World Health Organisation revealed that consuming 25-29 grams of fibre a day decreases the risk of heart disease, stroke, type 2 diabetes and bowel cancer as well as of dying early from heart disease - or indeed from any other cause - by 15–30 per cent. The report – a series of systematic reviews and meta-analyses, considered pretty much top of the heap when it comes to evidence – also found that those eating the highest fibre diets had a lower risk of overweight, high cholesterol, high blood pressure and breast cancer. Nuts and seeds, of course, along with fruit, vegetables, pulses and wholegrains, are a great source of fibre, which gets fermented by our gut bacteria to produce those secondary chemicals now thought to be so important for keeping a lid on disease.

FROM FARM TO FORK AND BEYOND

As plant foods, the nutrient value and potential health benefits of nuts and seeds don't just depend on the nutrients they contain. They also rely on a host of factors – some of which are in our control and some of which aren't. These include the soil in which they are grown, the climate, their exposure to stress (yes, plants get stressed too though by things such as lack of water or too much heat rather than being stuck in a traffic jam), as well as how they are harvested, transported, processed and stored, the form in which we eat them, and the way our bodies deal with them once they hit our digestive system.

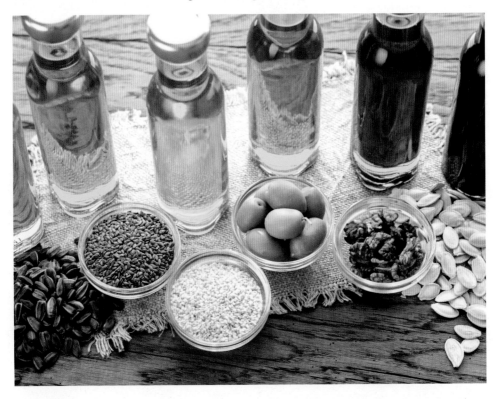

NUTS AND SEEDS

Once we take them home, whether we eat them whole, chopped, ground, raw, roasted or toasted, in oils or butters, as dairy-milk alternatives, sprouted and so on can all affect their nutrient value, digestibility and how they affect our body too. Roasting, for example, often boosts levels of polyphenols, but it may have less desirable effects on other nutrients – again a good reason to vary how you eat them. You'll find ideas and hints about how to prepare and use nuts and seeds for optimal health benefits as you read through the individual entries.

FROM CHECKOUT TO CUPBOARD

One thing to bear in mind is that the rich polyunsaturated fatty acid (PUFA) content of nuts and seeds means they are highly prone to turning rancid – aka oxidation. The good news is that they contain their own inbuilt antioxidants, such as vitamin E, that can help protect against this. But they won't last forever. So, for maximum freshness buy in small quantities and use quickly. Buying loose? Shop at a busy store that stocks up on fresh nuts often and, once home, store them at a constant temperature in a sealed, airtight container in a cool, dry cupboard, pantry, fridge or freezer.

Note: Let your senses be your guide. If nuts or seeds look dry, mouldy or discoloured, smell or taste unpleasant, bitter, or less than fresh, ditch them. Shell-on nuts will keep the longest and processed nuts e.g. halved, skinned, chopped or ground, the shortest length of time.

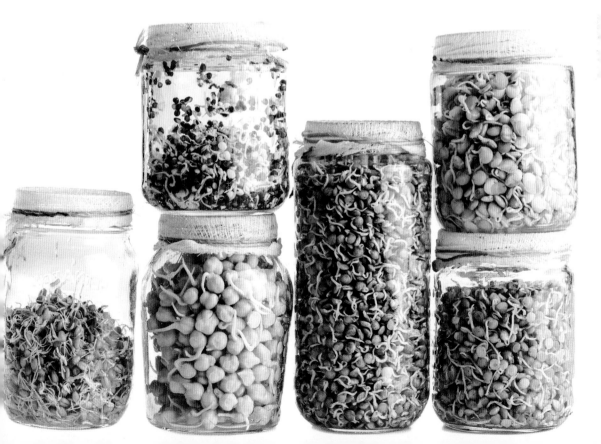

Check below to see how long after the use-by or best before date various nuts and seeds will keep...

Nuts	Cupboard/Pantry	Fridge	Freezer
Almonds	9-12	12	24
Brazils	9	12	12
Cashews	6-9	12	24
Hazels	4-6	12	24
Macadamias	6-9	12	24
Peanuts	6-9	12	24
Peanut butter (smooth or crunchy)	12	12	N/a
Peanut butter (natural)	2-3	3-6	N/a
Pecans	6	12	24
Pine nuts	1-2	3-4	5-6
Pistachios	3	3	12
Walnuts	6	12	24
Seeds	Cupboard/Pantry	Fridge	Freezer
Chia (seeds)	Up to 24	48+	48+
Chia (milled)	2-4 weeks	12-24	12-24
Flax (seeds)	6-12	12	12
Flax (milled)	1 weeks	1-2	1-2
Hemp (seeds)	6-12	12	12
Hemp (milled)	1 week	1-2	1-2
Pumpkin	2-3	12	12
Sesame (seeds)	6-12	12	12
Sesame (roasted)	12-36	12-36	12-36
Sesame (tahini paste)	4-6	4-6	4-6
Sunflower (raw)	2-3	12	12
Sunflower (roasted shelled)	3-4	12	12
Sunflower (roasted shell-on)	4-5	12	12
Sunflower butter	6	6	N/a
Quinoa (white, red or black)	24-36	24-36	N/a

All storage times in months unless otherwise specified.

SPROUTING

Incidentally one way to boost the nutrient value of seeds as well as their digestibility is to sprout or germinate them. Doing so can reduce their carbohydrate and boost their protein content as well as increasing levels of vitamins such as vitamin C and making some minerals such as iron and zinc more bioavailable, that is better able to be used by our cells.

It can also increase their polyphenol content as a 2018 study in the journal *Food Chemistry* showed. It found that the polyphenol content of hemp seeds was considerably enhanced when they were sprouted for three to five days. Sprouted seeds are great added to salads, sandwiches, popped in smoothies or used to top bakes, soups and other dishes. You can sprout them in a jar with a pierced lid or piece of gauze or hessian or take the sweat out of it by investing in a special germinator or sprouting jar.

SOAK AWAY

Precise soaking and sprouting times vary from seed to seed but as a general rule of thumb here's how:

1. Place seeds in the container (fill it up no more than a third to allow space for the sprouted seeds).
2. Cover with water and soak overnight before rinsing and draining.
3. Keep the container somewhere dark and repeat the rinsing and draining process at least once every 12 hours until the seeds have fully sprouted – usually about 2 to 4 days.
4. Drain well, rinse again and store them in the fridge – they will usually keep for two or three days.

Note: Sprouted seeds can cause food poisoning so always rinse and don't keep longer than two or three days. Discard the seeds if they brown or change colour. Certain people are more vulnerable to food poisoning and should not eat raw sprouted seeds. These include older people, the very young, pregnant women and anyone with a weakened immune system due to underlying health issues.

NUTS, SEEDS AND FAKE NEWS

Just before we put the individual nuts and seeds under the microscope, a word or two about those media stories many of which, frankly, fall into the category of fake news. This usually comes about as a result of reporting studies piecemeal and picking the ones that make for the most headline-grabbing story, no matter that it was just done in cells, in a test tube or in mice. Now, as a rule, what editors want is surprising or counter-intuitive stories. Think of the old news desk dictum, 'If a dog bites a man it isn't news, but if a man bites a dog it is.' Science on the other hand – bar the odd true breakthrough or happy accident – is mainly about doing something and then doing it again to see if the same result can be achieved.

The thing is – and it's why scientists and journalists often regard each other with mutual suspicion – although science never stands still, it tends to evolve rather than progress in leaps and bounds. So it's not the newest, quirkiest finding that counts, but the one that's the most convincing, given the quality of the research, and the total weight of all the evidence put together.

Studies done in a test tube and the likes of fruit flies, worms, rats and mice, can help set scientists on the path to further exploration or throw light on the mechanics of what happens when a particular food or nutrient gets into the body, though bear in mind that these creatures aren't people and results don't always carry across. So too can those 'observational' studies, which look for links between certain foods or diets and particular diseases as well as small 'pilot' trials in people.

But as every science student gets drummed into them, 'Correlation does not equal cause' – meaning that just because two things are linked, one doesn't necessarily result in the other. It's only by doing clinical trials and looking at the large overviews we call systematic reviews and meta-analyses that roll up all the evidence to reach a conclusion that we can really decide if a proposition stands up.

If you want to find out more about how to judge those media stories turn to page 126 to read about this 'hierarchy of evidence'. It's not perfect, especially in a science like nutrition where we're dealing with humans and their messy lives, unreliable memories, and haphazard eating habits rather than cells, or lab animals whose diet and living conditions can be controlled. But, hopefully, it will help you decide how seriously to take it next time you see a headline claiming that this or that food does or doesn't cause heart disease, cancer or dementia.

In the rest of this book we'll be looking at some popular nuts and seeds in turn to discover what's so healthy about them. But before we do that, it's worth stressing once more that we don't eat foods in isolation – and we certainly don't eat nutrients – they are part of the rich and complex mix that makes up our overall diet. So, if you don't like a particular nut or seed, all you have to do is choose a different variety and make it part of your eating pattern.

ALMONDS

Prunus dulcis

Adding almonds to your diet could help boost heart and brain health, control blood glucose and protect against type 2 diabetes as well as helping you reach and remain a healthy weight, maintain good digestive health, and fend off infections.

Native to areas of the Middle East with a Mediterranean climate, almonds were probably first cultivated in the early Bronze Age some 4,000-5,000 years ago. Some 3,000 years later and almonds – and watermelon seeds – were packed into the tomb of the Egyptian pharaoh, Tutankhamun. Today the rest of the world has cottoned on to the delights of almonds and they still go down a treat in the Middle East and Mediterranean.

Almonds are among the nuts included in that great study of the benefits of a Mediterranean Diet, the PREDIMED Study (see page 120). And, given their nutrient profile, it's not surprising. With the highest protein content of any tree nut, almonds also contain the monounsaturated fatty acid (MUFA), oleic acid, also found in olive

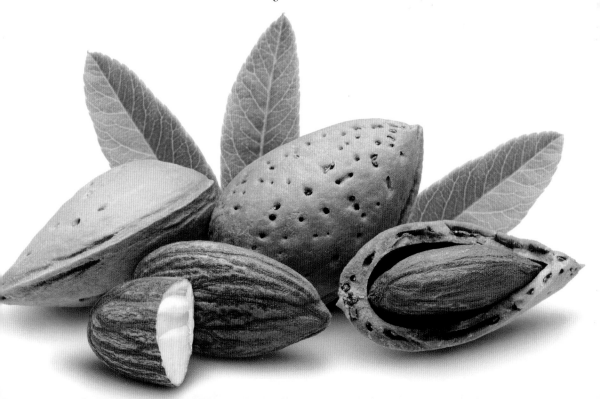

oil, polyunsaturated fatty acids (PUFAs) as well as having some of the highest levels among tree nuts of calcium and magnesium. Almond skins meanwhile are rich in fibre and abound in health promoting polyphenols. And that's just for starters. Let's drill down a bit deeper into those potential health benefits.

WEIGHT AND WAIST

If you're worried that putting almonds on the menu will lead to a bulging waistline, you might want to think again in the light of a study of overweight and obese adults, published in the *International Journal of Obesity and Related Metabolic Disorders*. The participants, 65 in all, aged between 27 and 79 years, either went on a low-calorie 'shakes and soups' slimming diet with 84 grams of pre-packed whole, unblanched, unsalted almonds as a snack, or a self-chosen diet with exactly the same amount of energy and protein based around complex carbohydrates – think things like wholegrains, pulses, wholemeal bread and pasta– plus safflower oil for fat.

At the end of the study, which lasted 24 weeks, those on the almond- enriched diet had lost 62per cent more weight and seen their waist circumference shrink by 50per cent more than those on the complex carb diet. And they also saw a 56per cent reduction in the amount of fat stored in their bodies.

What's especially interesting about this study is that those on the almond-enriched diet got 39per cent of their calories from fat and 32per cent from carbs. Those in the other group, meanwhile, got just 18per cent of calories from fat but 53per cent from those complex carbs. More to the point 25per cent of fats in the group who snacked on almonds were those heart-friendly MUFAs, while only 5per cent of fats in the complex carb diet came from MUFAs. It's a vivid illustration of how, despite eating a diet with the same calorie count, the source of those calories appears to make a difference to our vital statistics.

In another trial published in the *Journal of the American Heart Association*, participants who consumed a daily handful of almonds also saw a shrinkage in the fat around their waistline. Fat in this area – what scientists call central adiposity and the rest of us call middle-aged spread – is a tell-tale sign of 'visceral fat', a type of fat that accumulates around the vital organs, which is increasingly being recognised as a risk factor for diseases such as type 2 diabetes, heart disease and stroke.

TYPE 2 DIABETES

Now it can't have escaped your notice that type 2 diabetes, which is linked to overweight and obesity, has reached epidemic proportions throughout the Western world. It happens when the hormone insulin, which helps keep blood glucose steady, stops working properly. Eventually, after trying to right this, the pancreas, which produces insulin, gives up, causing soaring blood glucose levels. So, anything that can help lower blood glucose levels and help quell hunger pangs is worth a try.

In a study published in the *European Journal of Clinical Nutrition* participants with a high risk of type 2 diabetes snacked on 43 grams of almonds a day, either as an accompaniment to breakfast or lunch or as a morning or afternoon snack. The study revealed that this helped to lower levels of blood glucose with the findings being most marked in those who consumed them as a snack. And that's not all. Snacking on almonds also helped curb hunger. Even better news, in common with other studies on nuts, there was no evidence that those almond snacks led to weight gain. It seems that study participants automatically reduced their calorie intake to make up for the extra calories supplied by the almonds.

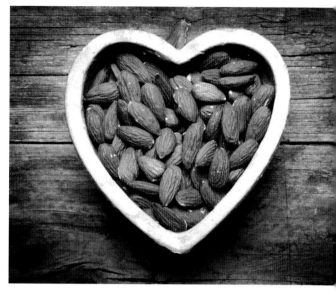

HEART

And so to the heart, where studies suggest that almonds can help lower classic 'markers' of cardiovascular disease such as high levels of 'bad' LDL cholesterol. Here too it seems almonds score, according to a handful of studies. One published in *Nutrition Research and Practice* found that an almond snack between meals was one of the best ways to attain a healthy blood fat profile. Meanwhile according to a second study in the *Journal of the American Heart Association,* a daily handful of almonds (42 grams a day) as part of an overall cholesterol-lowering diet, lowered levels of 'bad' LDL cholesterol, while maintaining levels of 'good' HDL cholesterol compared to an identical diet with an added muffin but no almonds.

The good news is these benefits seem to apply whether you are healthy or already have a diagnosis of heart disease or related problems. In one study, published in the *Journal of Nutrition,* for example, researchers asked 150 men and women diagnosed with heart disease to eat just 10 grams a day of almonds before breakfast, a step that boosted 'good' HDL cholesterol as well as improving other aspects of blood fat profile. Almonds could even prove a useful extra if you already take statins to help lower cholesterol, according to a study in the *Journal of Clinical Lipidology.* Statin users had significantly lower levels of 'bad' LDL cholesterol after just four weeks of eating a daily 100 grams of almonds– useful to know if you are taking statins.

The reason for these beneficial effects? Key candidates are those heart-friendly MUFAs and PUFAs as well as fibre and phytosterols – all nutrients that may help us to a healthier blood fat profile. But that's not all. Almonds also contain a cocktail of other nutrients, including vitamin E, and the minerals, magnesium, copper, manganese, calcium, and potassium, plus a plant-form of the amino acid, arginine, which is needed to produce nitric oxide a compound that helps keep arteries elastic.

BRAIN

Back in the day, most research on the benefits of almonds focused, like most research on nuts, mainly on their effects on the heart and blood vessels. But as we're all getting older and more and more of us are developing dementia the spotlight has turned towards the brain. And it's now recognised that 'What is good for the heart is good for the brain.'

A review published in the journal *Pharmacological Research*, highlights the potential benefits of almonds, hazelnuts and walnuts to protect the brain and defend against Alzheimer's disease. Their secret? Researchers point to brain-friendly nutrients such as oleic acid, which encourages the growth of brain cells, as well as the omega-6 fatty acid, linoleic acid, which may help protect brain cells against damage.

Almond skins are also a source of fibre and those polyphenol plant chemicals which, according to this review, are linked with better memory, the production of new brain cells and prevention of brain cell death. It's early days yet, of course, and research on the potential brain benefits of almonds is still scarce but it's certainly a promising start.

INFECTIONS

But this isn't the end of the almond story. Some studies now suggest that polyphenols found in almond skins could help combat infections, a useful asset in a world in which antibiotic resistance is increasing and new ways to fight infection are thin on the ground.

In an early test-tube study, published in *Letters in Microbiology*, researchers discovered that polyphenol-rich almond skin extracts were active against the two food poisoning bugs, listeria and salmonella, as well as several other disease-causing agents and the fungus candida albicans.

Research published in *Molecules*, meanwhile, found that almond skin extracts blocked a family of inflammatory chemicals and triggered the release of anti-inflammatory chemicals in cells infected by herpes simplex virus-2 (HSV-2), which causes genital herpes. In other research by the same team published in the journal *Viruses*, almond skin extracts stopped the herpes simplex virus-1 (HSV-1) responsible for cold sores

> ### GOOD NEWS FOR CHOCOLATE LOVERS
>
> According to a US study in the *Journal of the American Heart Association*, people who consumed 42.5 grams a day of almonds together with 18 grams a day of cocoa powder and 43 grams a day of dark chocolate saw a greater reduction in small, dense 'bad' LDL cholesterol particles, which experts now think are especially harmful for artery health.

from sticking to cells, so preventing them from replicating. All most intriguing and a further reminder when shopping for almonds to choose them in their skins.

CANCER

So what about that other scourge of twenty-first-century life: cancer? There's really not much research to go on here. But what there is hints at potential benefit, such as this Mexican study published in *Biologic and Gynaecologic Investigation*. The researchers examined the diets of 97 women with breast cancer and 104 women without the disease and what they found was thought provoking. Women who, over the course of their lives, had eaten a diet rich in almonds, peanuts or walnuts, had a two to threefold lower risk of breast cancer. Caution is needed here of course. Their nut consumption could simply reflect a healthier diet overall. This was just one small study and, a link between two factors doesn't necessarily point to a causal link. Nevertheless it is interesting.

There is also a clue that almond oil, long used in traditional medicine, could help keep the bowel healthy. According to a Turkish study published in *Pharmaceutical Biology*, almond oil from Northern Cyprus and Turkey helped curb the proliferation of colon cancer cells and, suggest the researchers, may have anti-cancer properties. Again it's one small study, and a lab one at that. However it's an area of research worth keeping an eye on.

GUT

Of course, in nutrition it's all about the gut these days or more precisely, the gut microbiome, the community of bacteria and other microorganisms that inhabits our

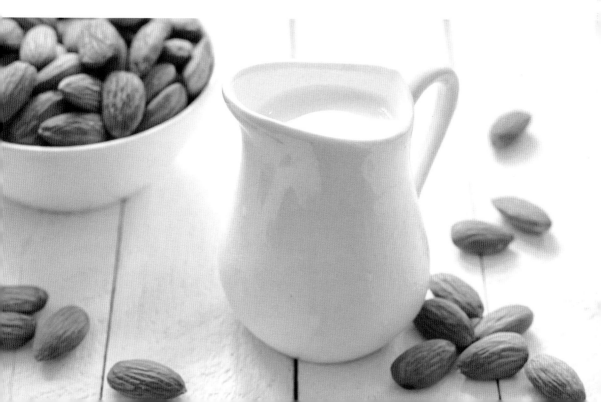

large intestine. So a study in the *British Journal of Nutrition* is especially tantalising. It seems that almonds – and especially their fibre-rich skins – pass undigested into the large intestine or bowel where they ferment and encourage the growth of healthy bacteria. In other words they act as 'prebiotics', fermentable foods or food ingredients that help to gut bacteria to flourish in a way that's similar to how garden soil rich in organic matter helps plants to grow.

And the benefits may not stop there. When Italian researchers added natural almond skin powder to the food of mice with the inflammatory bowel disease (IBD), colitis, they – the mice that is – suffered far less with diarrhoea and weight loss, two of the most debilitating symptoms of IBD, as well as producing fewer inflammatory chemicals. As so often, it's early days yet to draw firm conclusions, but it's yet another hint that almonds could be a good thing for the gut.

IN THE KITCHEN

Sprinkle chopped, toasted almonds over porridge made with oats or other grains such as millet or quinoa.

Add whole or flaked almonds to curries, stews and tagines. Ground almonds are a key ingredient of the popular Kashmiri lamb curry, rogan josh.

Replace dairy milk in tea, coffee, sauces and desserts with almond drink. Almond drink also makes a good base for smoothies and protein shakes.

Snack on almonds – raw or roasted – between meals instead of cakes and biscuits.

Use almond oil in salad dressings.

Spread almond butter on oatcakes for a satisfying mid-morning or afternoon snack, or add a dollop to protein shakes and smoothies to boost nutritional value.

Dip whole almonds in melted dark chocolate and serve with strawberries or other berries for an extra polyphenol boost.

Get baking. Adding whole, ground skin-on almonds to bread, buns or biscuits could help boost the 'bioavailability' of plant nutrients found in almond skins.

YOUR CHOICE... To max out almonds' nutrient benefits, dry roast whole in their skins. Roasting almond kernels for 20 minutes at 200°C significantly boosts levels of antioxidant polyphenol plant compounds. In fact, the total polyphenol content in roasted almonds is around double that of blanched, freeze-dried almonds, according to research.

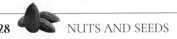

NUTS AND SEEDS

BRAZIL NUTS

Bertholletia excelsa

—

With the highest levels of the antioxidant trace element, selenium, of any nut plus protein, fibre, good fats, minerals and a range of plant chemicals, this three-sided nut in its rough dark shell could have the potential to improve the health of several organs, including the brain, heart, thyroid and more. Just don't eat too many!

Brazil nuts are seeds from the coconut-like fruit of the lofty tree which grows in the Amazonian rainforests. Native to – where else? – Brazil, as well as Bolivia and Peru, the nuts lie nestled inside the fruit, called *cosos* in Portuguese, arranged in segments, some twelve to twenty-four to each. Virtually all Brazil nuts consumed across the world come from wild trees rather than plantations. But curiously, Brazil nuts are not especially popular in their native land. This may be beginning to change, however, as several Brazilian research studies are revealing potential health benefits.

A CORNUCOPIA OF NUTRIENTS

Compared with other nuts, Brazil nuts contain more selenium, a 'trace' element present in soil and well-known for its antioxidant and anti-inflammatory properties.

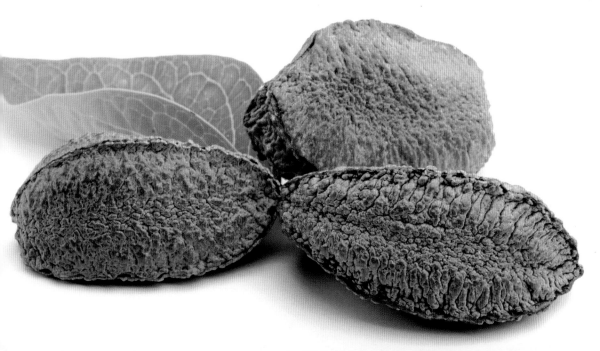

Several key enzymes in the body depend on selenium for activities from helping to keep the genetic material or DNA in our cells in good repair to optimum hormonal and immune function.

Although we only need a small amount of selenium – that's why it's called a 'trace' element – a deficiency of this mineral has been linked with an increased risk of cancer, heart disease, cognitive decline, and thyroid problems. But it is not just high selenium levels that make Brazil nuts unique it is also the quality of that selenium, which is extremely bioavailable – meaning it comes in a form that is easily absorbed and used by our bodies.

Like all nuts, Brazil nuts are also a source of MUFAs and PUFAs, including the plant omega-3, ALA – alpha-linolenic acid (see page 120). Brazil nuts contain rather more saturated fat than virtually any other nut except coconuts. And they also – along with almonds – have the highest concentration among tree nuts of those antioxidant polyphenols as well as plant sterols which may help reduce absorption of cholesterol plus another plant compound, squalene, a building block of hormones.

Lower in protein and carbohydrates than some other nuts, Brazil nuts have a similar fibre content to walnuts, and as well as selenium, contain another key antioxidant nutrient, vitamin E as well as higher concentrations of magnesium, copper and zinc than other nuts. With such credentials, how do they stack up on the health front?

HEART

Like other tree nuts, Brazil-nut consumption is linked with decreased risk of heart problems thanks to that wealth of nutrients. But what about selenium specifically, which they contain in such abundance? Research into the potential benefits of this trace mineral for the heart has been going on ever since the 1960s. So what has it found?

It certainly seems a shortage of selenium can increase the risk of heart disease. On the other hand, too much can harm the heart. On the plus side, according to a large Chinese review of studies published in the *European Journal of Nutrition*, selenium supplements can put a brake on inflammation and oxidative stress, both of which are thought to be involved in the development of cardiovascular conditions.

Could Brazil nuts have the same effect? To be honest, relatively few studies have examined this, and those there are have been small and somewhat contradictory. For example, one unrandomised Brazilian trial in *Nutrition Research* offers a hint that Brazil nuts could reduce the risk of heart disease. In this trial, thirty-seven women with serious weight problems who consumed just one Brazil nut a day saw an improvement in their levels of 'good' HDL cholesterol and a reduction in their risk of developing heart disease after just eight weeks. Clearly the findings of a study this small – and one with no control group to boot – is far from proof that Brazil nuts protect against heart disease, but it does give pause for thought.

Somewhat more convincing is another Brazilian study, published in *Nutrition and Metabolism* in which ten healthy individuals had their blood fats tested after consuming different amounts of Brazil nuts (specifically 0, 5, 20, or 50 grams). Six hours afterwards researchers detected a significant upturn in their blood levels of selenium; by the time nine hours had elapsed their levels of 'bad' LDL cholesterol were significantly lower and levels of 'good' HDL cholesterol were significantly higher, at least when they consumed 20 grams or 50 grams of nuts. This is good news because it suggests that even a single serving of Brazil nuts could improve blood fat profile in a relatively short time.

Another small Brazilian study of obese young teenage women, aged on average 15 years, found that eating the equivalent of three to five Brazil nuts a day reduced levels of 'bad' LDL cholesterol and triglycerides other blood fats implicated in heart disease as well as improving the function of tiny 'microvascular' blood vessels. The researchers surmise this was due to high level of PUFAs and other biologically active components that they do not specify.

It goes without saying that three small studies do not a benefit prove, something to bear in mind when considering the results of yet another study published in *Nutrition Research*. This found that 45 grams of Brazil nuts a day over the course of a fortnight didn't essentially change the blood fat profile of fifteen healthy people, even though the level of selenium in their blood rose. It did, however, slightly improve a pivotal chemical 'pathway' involved in transporting excess cholesterol back to the liver to be disposed of in the bile and eventually in faeces. This pathway is called the 'nonatherogenic reverse cholesterol transport pathway', a bit of a mouthful but a possible clue as to how Brazil nuts might work in favour of the heart.

What could account for these contradictions? Researchers are increasingly looking to the effects of our individual genetic makeup on differences in the way nutrients affect us, and an intriguing study published in the *European Journal of Nutrition* throws light on this. In the study, which involved 130 healthy men and women aged between 20 and 60 years, participants were asked to eat just one Brazil nut a day for eight weeks followed by eight

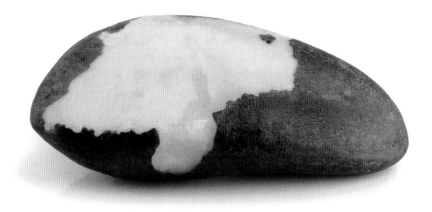

further weeks with no Brazil nuts and the Brazil nuts did indeed improve the blood fat profile of participants as well as lowering their blood glucose levels.

The next thing was to find out if the participants genetic makeup affected these findings so they checked out their DNA. Sure enough, even though Brazil nuts lowered cholesterol levels in all participants, they didn't do this as effectively in those with a certain kind of genetic variation – what scientists call a SNP (pronounced snip). It's a fascinating finding and one that points towards a future in which we may all be able to tweak our diets in accordance with our individual genetic makeup, something called personalised nutrition. That day isn't yet here, but it isn't that far off.

BRAIN

Oxidative stress, cell damage caused by rogue molecules called oxygen free radicals, is thought to be a factor behind the lapses in attention and concentration and struggles with memory – aka cognitive impairment – that affect some of us as we get older. Could selenium help to counteract this? If the results of a small study in *the European Journal of Nutrition,* hold true it seems it could. This found eating just one Brazil nut a day for six months resulted in a significant improvement in verbal fluency, which measures how fast we can retrieve words from memory, as well as better performance other brain power tests. Not much to go on it's true but worth keeping an eye out to see if other studies back this up.

THYROID

Selenium – along with iodine and other micronutrients – is involved in the production of hormones produced by the thyroid, that butterfly-shaped gland in the neck whose hormones are needed by every single cell in the body. Thyroid problems, especially Hashimoto's thyroiditis, a key cause of underactivity of the thyroid gland (hypothyroidism) caused by an immune attack on the thyroid gland, tend to become more common as we get older, especially in women. And this has been linked to an inadequate intake of selenium.

An underactive thyroid (hypothyroidism) can lead to symptoms such as tiredness and fatigue, dry skin and hair, insomnia, depression, joint aches and pains, problems with concentration and oversensitivity to cold. Studies carried out in the 1990s suggest that low levels of selenium, especially in older people, are linked with lower levels of thyroid hormones and faulty thyroid function. The thyroid story is a complicated one, however, and iodine, as well as other micronutrients including iron, zinc and vitamin A, are all part of it. What these studies underline is the importance of eating a varied diet which provides a good mix of nutrients including those vital trace elements.

 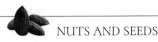

CANCER

What about cancer? Could Brazil nuts help to combat its development? The picture is currently not very clear – partly as a result of the variable quality and limitations of many studies. However, according to a large review published in January 2018 the incidence of certain types of cancer – for example stomach, bowel, lung, breast, bladder and prostate – as well as the risk of dying from cancer, is lowest in people with the highest blood levels of selenium.

As the researchers point out, not all studies are in accord, and unfortunately there is no clear cut pattern. Intriguingly though it does appear that, just as we saw with cholesterol and blood glucose levels, selenium may help modify cancer risk in people with genetic variations in certain antioxidant enzymes. As so often, we need to know more before drawing conclusions.

And that's about it, apart from one small pilot study published in the *British Journal of Nutrition* which did examine the potential benefits of Brazil nuts for cancer prevention. This found that consuming six Brazil nuts a day for six weeks increased blood levels of selenium and had beneficial effects on chemical 'pathways' involved in the development of bowel cancer. While the researchers attributed this to the selenium in Brazil nuts they surmise that other plant chemicals in Brazils could be part of the picture.

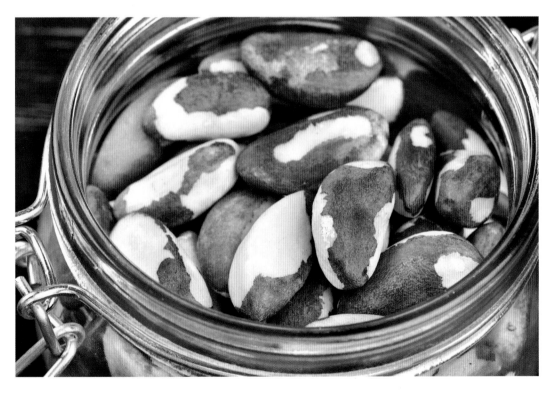

TOO MUCH OF A GOOD THING?

Before we leave Brazil nuts, however, a few words of warning. When it comes to selenium it is vital not to overdo it. The reason? In the right amount selenium has potentially valuable antioxidant effects. At high levels, however, it can act as a pro-oxidant – that is it can increase the damaging effects of oxidative stress on the body's cells and increase the risk of health problems.

Experts are still arguing about the pros and cons. But, given the potentially high levels of selenium in Brazil nuts – from 0.03–512 milligrams – depending on where they have been grown, it is possible to overdose. To be on the safe side it's probably best not to eat too many Brazil nuts, just two a week is plenty according to one expert. Having more than this from time to time is unlikely to do you any harm, however, as long as you're not scoffing handfuls every day. So, bearing this in mind here are some ideas for ways to use them – occasionally!

IN THE KITCHEN

Process in a food processor with a handful of basil, lemon zest and olive oil for a different take on pesto.

Add a couple of chopped Brazil nuts to biscuits made with other nuts such as almonds or hazelnuts.

Slip a spoonful of ground Brazil nuts into humous.

Grate Brazil nuts on the fine side of the grater and use to top dips, salads or soups.

Chop one or two Brazil nuts and add to homemade nut butters made from other nuts to add a little crunch.

Add to fruit cakes such as the British traditional Christmas cake and/or glaze with honey or apricot jam and use to top fruit cakes with candied fruit.

Dip them in melted dark chocolate for an after dinner treat.

CASHEW NUTS

Anacardium occidentale

A great source of heart-healthy MUFAs and PUFAs, cashews also contain saturated fat, protein and fibre, plus antioxidant vitamins, such as beta-carotene, a precursor of vitamin A, B vitamins, two forms of vitamin E, and minerals including potassium, phosphorus, magnesium, calcium, iron, zinc and selenium. They are also rich in biologically active plant chemicals including cholesterol-lowering plant sterols all of which could benefit the heart and other areas of health.

The Portuguese discovered cashews in north-east Brazil back in the sixteenth century and brought them to Europe, since when they have spread to Africa, India and south-east Asia. Although they are called nuts, cashews are in fact the seeds of a tall, evergreen tree. This produces soft, shiny, juicy fruit known as cashew apples (actually swollen stems) much prized for their juice in Brazil, where they can be found on sale at roadside stalls packed into egg boxes. In the West, however, where cashew juice is virtually unknown, it is the soft, kidney shaped seeds that dangle, each in its own hard, greyish shell, from the bottom of the fruit, that rate highest in the snack stakes.

Surprisingly, though, despite ranking third in the global nut production league table, research on the potential health benefits of cashews is sparse. The reason for this is perhaps their relatively high saturated fat content which, has raised doubts about the wisdom of recommending them for regular consumption.

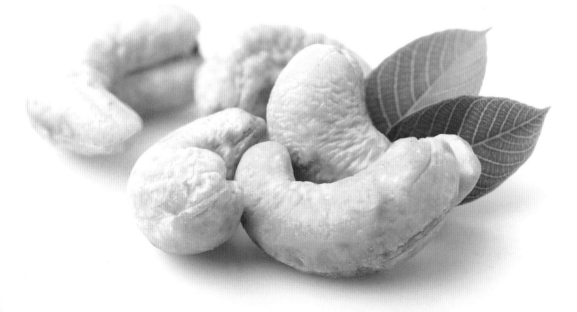

HEART

Cashew nuts are especially rich in the MUFA, oleic acid, the main fat in olive oil, which has been linked with a lower risk of cardiovascular problems. And although they also contain saturated fats, the main one of these is stearic acid, which is thought to be fairly neutral in its effects on cholesterol. Despite this, cashews haven't usually been recommended for heart health. This could be about to change thanks to two randomised, controlled trials.

In the first, published in the *American Journal of Clinical Nutrition*, fifty-one men and women aged 21 to 73 swapped potato crisps for cashew nuts at snack time. At the end of the study blood sampling revealed that both their total and 'bad' LDL cholesterol levels had taken a downturn – even though apart from this simple swap they hadn't changed anything else in their diet. A small study, it's true, but one that nevertheless suggests that choosing a handful of cashews over a high-calorie, high carb snack, could be a pretty effortless way to push those cholesterol levels in the right direction.

The second trial, published in the *Journal of Nutrition* looked at the effects of cashew nuts on the heart health of people with type 2 diabetes, a disease that pushes up the risk of heart problems. It was carried out in India, a country with an especially high incidence of type 2 diabetes and cardiovascular disease and included 300 people with diabetes from the city of Chennai on the Bay of Bengal.

The participants, aged between 30 and 65 years, were divided into two groups and randomly allotted to eat either the standard diet recommended for people with diabetes or the same diet with an added 30 grams of raw, unsalted cashew nuts daily. Both groups stuck with their usual activity and medication regimens. At the end of the study, which lasted just twelve weeks, those who had added cashew nuts to the menu had experienced a drop in systolic blood pressure (BP). This is the upper BP number which reflects the pressure in our arteries when the heart contracts, so a lower

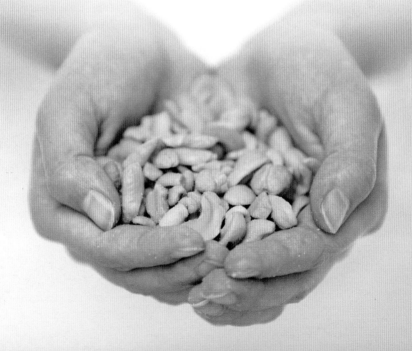

reading is a good thing. And the participants who ate cashew nuts also experienced a rise in 'good' HDL cholesterol.

Meanwhile, in accord with studies of other nuts, even though the group who added cashew nuts to their diet consumed more calories, they didn't gain weight or inches around the waist. A great result that suggests snacking on a few cashews could be a good move – and certainly better than reaching for the biscuit tin.

What could account for these findings? We already know about the fatty acid content of cashew nuts. But that's not the end of the story. They also contain protein, fibre, vitamin E, the mineral potassium, which is needed for healthy blood pressure plus several plant chemicals including plant sterols, natural compounds similar to cholesterol which, say studies, can help to lower both total and 'bad' LDL cholesterol.

OTHER HEALTH BENEFITS

Could cashews benefit health in other ways? There are so few specific studies that it's hard to say. However, we do know that they contain a range of polyphenols, in amounts similar to those found in green beans, spinach, blueberries and apples, all known for their potential health effects.

More specifically cashews have levels of lignans, fibre-linked plant chemicals that help promote healthy gut bacteria associated with protection against heart disease, hormone-linked cancers and osteoporosis. The amounts in cashew nuts are similar to those in flax and sesame seeds, the main food sources for lignans. All of this suggests that, although it's not possible to make any firm recommendations, you could certainly do worse than having a handful of cashews as a snack or spreading a slick of cashew nut butter on your morning toast from time to time.

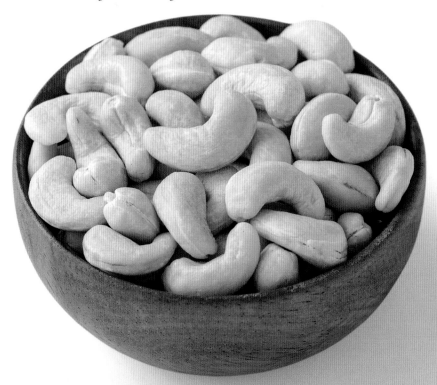

IN THE KITCHEN

Combine raw cashews with other nuts and/or seeds or dried fruits in snacks or trail mixes.

Add whole cashews or cashew nut butter to stir-fries, Indian-style curries and south-east Asian dishes – they are especially good ground with almonds and raisins to make a paste in Kashmiri style curries such as Kashmiri Murgh Marsala.

Sprinkle untoasted cashews over salads dressed with sesame oil, soy sauce, lime juice, garlic and ginger.

Add chopped cashews to sweet or savoury flapjacks.

Spread a dollop of cashew butter on toast or crackers and/or add to breakfast smoothies.

Place cashews on a baking sheet and roast at around 75°C (160–170°F) for 15–20 minutes and eat as a snack. For a savoury take, roll in a little soy sauce before roasting.

DID YOU KNOW?

A relative of mango, pistachio and poison ivy, cashews used to be known as 'blister nuts'. Why? The shells contain a poisonous oil, urushiol, also known as cashew balm, which causes an itchy, red, blistering rash. This is why, unlike other tree nuts, you won't find them whole in their shells.

IT'S YOUR CHOICE...

High-temperature dry roasting doubles the ability of cashew kernels to mop up free radicals, those rogue molecules that can damage cells. Way to go if you want to enhance the antioxidant activity of plant chemicals in cashew nuts.

CHIA SEEDS

Salvia hispanica

Once confined to the shelves of health stores, the tiny seeds of this ancient grain, a member of mint family, are hailed in headlines as a 'superfood' and are all over Instagram and other social media platforms in breakfast bowls, smoothies, puddings and cakes. But is there any truth behind the hype?

Chia has featured on the human menu for some 5,500 years. Indeed, in pre-historic times it was second only to beans as a staple crop and the Aztecs and the Mayans used it in food, medicines, cosmetics and religious ceremonies. Today you'll find chia seeds on sale as whole seeds or powders and as ingredients in 'functional foods' from energy bars to cereals, yoghurts, breads and energy drinks.

One of the things that sets chia seeds apart from other seeds is their PUFA – polyunsaturated fatty acid –content. Around 65 per cent of this is a plant form of the omega-3 PUFA, ALA – aka alpha-linolenic acid, and they also contain omega-6 PUFAs. Is it any wonder that the word 'chia' comes from the Spanish 'chian' meaning oily? Chia seeds actually have the highest percentage per gram of any plant food of ALA. Combine this with a high protein content, a good helping of fibre, vitamins and minerals, including calcium, iron, magnesium, phosphorus and potassium and an array of natural antioxidant plant compounds, and it's not surprising they have such a stellar reputation. But what does the research say – and what could it mean for you?

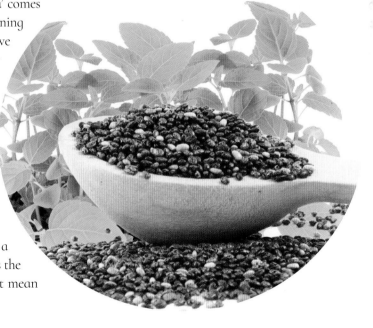

HEART

With their high ALA content chia seeds are often advanced as candidates for helping heart health. And, although not as effective as long chain omega-3 PUFAs found in oily fish, which come in a form our bodies find easier to use, it does seem that ALA could help lower levels of 'bad' LDL cholesterol and increase levels of 'good' HDL cholesterol. So, if you are vegetarian, vegan or don't like fish and don't get that one portion of oily fish a week recommended for health, then chia seeds could be worth putting on the menu.

But the potential benefits of chia seeds don't only depend on their oil content. They also contain a variety of types of vitamin E. They are exceptionally high in different types of fibre too – between 34 and 40 grams per 100 grams higher than quinoa, flaxseed, and amaranth. It is this high fibre content – and in particular the gluey, gelatinous stuff sometimes known as soluble fibre – that makes them such an asset when added to smoothies, breakfast bowls and desserts. How? It gives chia seeds the ability to swell to around ten times their dry weight in liquid.

So, do chia seeds enhance cardiovascular health? Well rats and rabbits whose food has added chia oil, milled or whole seeds certainly have a better blood fat profile. But does this carry over to humans? So far, unfortunately the evidence is rather more scarce.

A small Brazilian study of twenty-six middle-aged men and women, for example, published in a journal called *Nutricia Hospitalaria* found that including 35 grams of chia flour a day in the diet for twelve weeks did lower total cholesterol and very low density lipoprotein (VLDL), an especially harmful kind of cholesterol where the arteries are concerned. It also increased levels of 'good' HDL cholesterol. However, this applied only in people with a poor blood fat profile to begin with. So, if you're healthy and hoping to improve your cholesterol profile by including chia seeds in your diet, they may not have much effect. Then again, this was a small study so perhaps we can't draw too many conclusions.

More promising, at first sight, is a report in *Diabetes Care* in which eleven men and nine women with type 2 diabetes took either around 37 grams of chia seeds or the same amount of wheat bran for twelve weeks. At the end of this time those who had taken chia seeds had lower systolic blood pressure (BP) and lower levels of

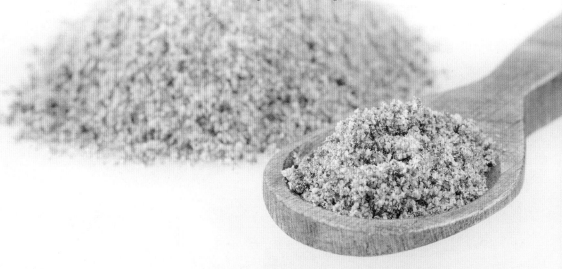

inflammatory chemicals as well as a slimmer waist circumference, body mass index and other potential risk factors for heart disease.

The trouble is, as well as being only a small study, this one was what scientists call 'single blinded', meaning that although participants don't know whether they were taking chia or bran, the researchers did, which of course can potentially bias results. The gold standard for studies is randomised and 'double blinded', meaning that neither researchers nor participants know who is taking a potentially active ingredient.

What's more, other research contradicts these potentially positive results. For instance, in one study in the journal *Nutrition Research* consuming 50 grams of chia seeds a day had *no* effect on body mass or fat levels, or markers of heart-disease risk such as inflammation, oxidative stress, blood pressure, and blood fats. So, on the heart health front at least, while chia seeds look promising, the jury is still out.

WAIST AND APPETITE

What about weight control, one of the other much-hyped qualities of chia seeds? In the study already mentioned, chia seeds were linked with a slimmer waist as well as with lower levels of C-reactive protein, a chemical marker of inflammation. We know that visceral fat, the sort that gathers around organs, produces inflammation, so that is a potentially positive result. Another finding which could point to a role for chia seeds in helping to reduce visceral fat is this: the researchers measured a protein produced in fat called adiponectin, low levels of which are thought to be a possible culprit in many of the negative effects of visceral fat, those in the chia group had higher levels suggesting that they had less visceral fat.

So, given the usual caveats about small studies, it is possible that chia seeds could help in the quest to slim your waist and control weight. And here's a possible reason. In small study published in the *European Journal of Clinical Nutrition* researchers compared the effects of chia and flaxseeds on blood glucose and satiety – that feeling of fullness that helps stabilise energy levels and keeps us going from one meal to the next, this time in fifteen healthy people. The result? Chia seeds helped stabilise blood glucose and increased satiety, a finding that could come down to their fibre content, which helps to keep blood glucose levels steady and prevent spikes.

So, while both chia seeds and flaxseeds may benefit blood glucose control and satiety, it seems chia seeds may just have the edge, meaning that, if you're watching your waistline adding some chia seeds to the mix could possibly be a good choice. However, if you're looking for magic weight loss they are unlikely to help.

BONES

Chia seeds have a high calcium content – at 157 milligrams of calcium in a 25-gram portion of seeds this is more than the calcium in 100 millilitres of milk. They also contain boron which helps calcium to get into bones. As yet, however, there are no studies showing that chia seeds benefit bones, although as part of a healthy diet they could certainly contribute to your calcium intake.

WATCH THIS SPACE

Overall, however, it seems that when it comes to chia seeds, the hype is somewhat ahead of the science. And this was certainly born out in a recent review and meta-analysis published in *Nutrition Reviews*. In an examination of twelve trials of chia in healthy people with no medical problems, athletes, people with diabetes and those with the pre-diabetic metabolic syndrome the effects of chia seeds appear to be at best modest, although there were hints of benefits for blood glucose and blood pressure levels.

One intriguing finding from this review is that milled (ground) chia seeds could be more effective than the whole seeds, another example of how processing can make all the difference to the availability of nutrients. In this review milled chia seeds appeared more effective in reducing systolic BP, the top BP reading reflecting pressure in the arteries when the heart beats, and in lowering fasting blood glucose, and improving blood fat profile than whole chia seeds. However, whole chia seeds seemed to be better for lowering levels of blood glucose after meals. It's yet another example of why it's always a good idea to vary your diet and the way you consume foods.

It has to be said though, that overall the researchers assessed the quality of the studies as low or very low. So rather disappointing if you're a chia seeds fan, and a cautionary tale that underlines the importance of well-planned and carried out studies and of taking wild claims that appear in the headlines with a pinch of salt.

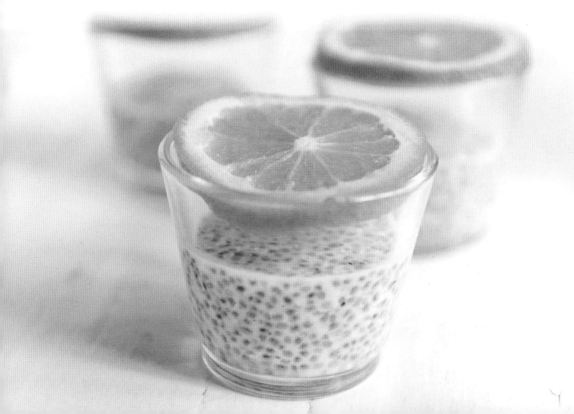

IN THE KITCHEN

Add a spoonful of whole or ground chia seeds to thicken smoothies, juices or breakfast bowls.

Mix them into yoghurt, kefir or oatmeal for an added nutrient punch.

Sprinkle on salads, soups, casseroles and stews or add to dips.

Use to add fibre to bread and bakes.

Make chia-seed pudding, top with a slice of orange or other fruit – you'll find recipes on the internet.

Ring the changes in salad dressings by replacing other oils with chia seed oil – don't heat it however, as this destroys its nutrient properties.

IT'S YOUR CHOICE...

To maximise nutritional value, try sprouting chia seeds and look for sprouted chia seed powder. A recent study showed that germinating the seeds increased their antioxidant and other beneficial properties.

DID YOU KNOW?

If you have coeliac disease, chia seeds are gluten free. They could also be useful for those with allergies. A small study of the impact of chia on allergy found that it was well tolerated and had no adverse effects on skin, digestive system or behaviour, although check with your healthcare professional if you are an allergy sufferer.

FLAXSEEDS

Linum usitatissimum

Best known in the past as the basis of that painter's standby, linseed oil, or of the ubiquitous mid-twentieth century flooring, lino, in the twenty-first century, flaxseeds and their oil have undergone a reinvention and the reputation of these small, flat seeds has rocketed. Research suggests they could help protect against heart disease, improve digestion and more.

Flax is, in fact, one of the oldest cultivated plants, grown for at least 7,000 years. Linseed oil was one of the few oils allowed during fasts in medieval Russia and was used in pea dishes. Meanwhile in the seventeenth century it was used in fish dishes for the delectation of the Czar.

Today flaxseeds are known as being among the best sources of that plant omega-3 PUFA, ALA, plus fibre, protein and minerals such as manganese and magnesium. Flaxseeds are also the richest source of lignans, fibre-linked antioxidant plant chemicals similar to the hormone, oestrogen. In fact they contain 100 times more lignans than other sources such as wholegrains, sesame seeds, vegetables, and fruits. So what might be the positive effects of all these on health?

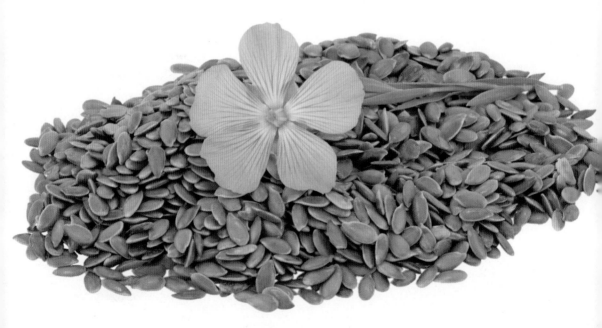

HEART

Flaxseeds' claimed benefits for heart health include lowering blood pressure, improving blood fat profile, combating oxidative stress, reducing inflammation, controlling blood glucose, helping reduce the tendency of blood to clot and helping to block irregular heart rhythms (arrhythmias). Let's start by looking at blood pressure in more detail.

As far as blood pressure is concerned you could certainly do worse than add a handful of ground flaxseeds to your morning breakfast cereal, according to Canadian researchers who looked at their effects on blood pressure in a group of people diagnosed with peripheral artery disease (PAD), furred, narrowed arteries in the arms and legs. Many of those studied had high blood pressure despite taking medication.

As well as high blood pressure and pain in the legs when walking, people with PAD usually have other risk factors for heart problems – think diabetes, high cholesterol, changes in blood clotting and furred, narrowed arteries. In the study, fifty-eight participants were issued with a variety of goodies – things like bagels, muffins, bars, buns, pasta, tea biscuits each containing 30g of ground flaxseed – and asked to eat one a day for six months. Fifty-two participants, meanwhile, who were identical in every other way to the first group were given the same food items but with milled wheat added instead of flaxseed.

The results, published in *Hypertension,* were hands down in favour of flaxseeds, with those in the flaxseed group experiencing an average fall of 10 millimetres of mercury in systolic BP, the top figure on the BP reading, the highest BP when the heart is beating to push blood around the body. They also experienced a drop of 7 millimetres of mercury in diastolic BP, the bottom figure, the lowest BP between heart beats. Meanwhile there was no difference, and sometimes even a rise in blood pressure readings, in the group given dummy foods. Better still, around 8 per cent of the flaxseed group being treated for high blood pressure were able to cut down on their medication. It may not sound a lot but it could make all the difference between having to take antihypertensive medications and not taking them or being able to reduce the dosage.

These results were confirmed in a later analysis of fifteen trials including 1,302 participants published in *Clinical Nutrition.* According to this, the most beneficial effects were seen after more than twelve weeks; in this analysis, ground flaxseed (flaxseed powder) was especially beneficial to systolic BP, which doctors consider the best indicator of the risk of having a stroke or heart attack. So it looks as though the best way to get the most out of flaxseeds is to put them in a grinder and give them a good whizz.

CHOLESTEROL

Flaxseeds also score on the cholesterol-lowering front according to an overview published in the *American Journal of Clinical Nutrition.* This found that flaxseeds lowered total and 'bad' LDL cholesterol with effects most pronounced in post-menopausal women and people with high cholesterol levels to begin with. Another small study from the *Journal of Nutrition*, meanwhile, found that a flax drink and a flax bread reduced total and 'bad' LDL-cholesterol by between 12 and 15 per cent in the case of the drink and 7 and 9 per cent in the case of the bread. It also increased the amount of fat passing out of the body in faeces. And in an arm of the Canadian study outlined above, ground flaxseed lowered both total and 'bad' LDL cholesterol as well as helping to reduce cholesterol in people who were taking anti-cholesterol medication. So all in all the case for putting flaxseeds on the menu to help improve cholesterol levels is looking pretty impressive.

INFLAMMATION

Experts are increasingly recognising that cholesterol levels are by no means the whole story when it comes to heart disease. In fact, it seems as if something has to happen in the arteries before cholesterol can worm its way into their lining; one of the key emerging players is inflammation so it is heartening to discover that, in rats at least, adding whole flaxseeds to a high-fat diet results in a remarkable reduction in inflammation.

But does the same apply to humans? The answer, it seems, is positive if you are obese – meaning you have a BMI of 30 or more – or are aged 50+. So says a research overview published in the journal *Nutrients*, which included more than 3,000 people. As so often, more research is needed, but it does point towards another potential benefit of adding flaxseeds to your diet.

DIABETES

There are also hints that flaxseeds may help control diabetes, according to a study by World Health Organisation scientists published in the *Journal of Dietary Supplements*. In the study eighteen people with type 2 diabetes added 10 grams of flaxseed powder

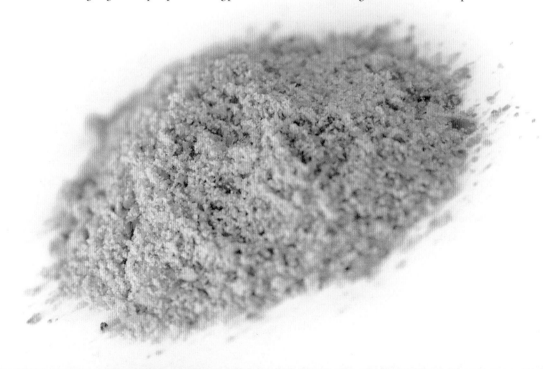

to their diet. Meanwhile a matched group did not do this. Apart from this, the diet and medication of both groups stayed the same. At the end of the study the blood glucose of those in the flaxseed group was almost 20 per cent lower, their overall blood glucose control was better, and they saw a reduction in blood fats.

This was only a small study, so while this is a promising result it's not enough to claim that flaxseeds can help manage type 2 diabetes. However it does make sense when you consider that, as a source of soluble fibre, flaxseeds help slow down the rate at which food passes out of the stomach so helping to prevent spikes in blood glucose. Lignans, those plant chemicals, which as we've seen are plentiful in flaxseeds, can also help reduce levels of blood glucose. Meanwhile the omega-3s may help improve the body's ability to deal with insulin and control blood sugar levels, according to a review published in the journal *Nutrition Reviews*. All in all, if you have type 2 diabetes or risk factors for diabetes, it looks as if flaxseeds could be ripe for inclusion on your menu.

GUT

Thanks to their high fibre content, flaxseeds have long had a reputation for helping digestion, easing constipation, and helping to protect against bowel diseases. But it is only recently, with the explosion of research into the gut, that researchers are starting to learn just how this may work. And the answer appears to be that they are changed by gut bacteria into so-called 'secondary' chemicals with benefits for health. The only drawback is that it seems not all of us have the right gut bacteria profile to do this, another example of how our genetic makeup may affect the way we use nutrients. What's more, most have been observed in animals rather than humans, and as you know this doesn't always translate across. But it's an interesting finding that certainly bears more investigation.

WEIGHT

Flaxseeds can help you feel fuller and curb appetite, which makes them useful if you're watching the pounds according to research published in the journal *Appetite*. But how do they do this? The answer again could lie in their effects on gut bacteria. One of the many benefits of healthy gut bacteria identified in recent years is weight control. So could this be their secret? A Danish study published in the *British Journal of Nutrition* suggests yes. Fifty-eight obese post-menopausal women took either a flaxseed supplement, a probiotic or a dummy pill.

After six weeks the flaxseed had kickstarted the women's insulin sensitivity – that is their ability to keep blood glucose levels stable. Insulin sensitivity has long been linked with lower weight and lower body fat as well as a lower risk of type 2 diabetes. They also had changes in their gut bacteria which were not seen in the women taking a probiotic. So could the effects of flaxseeds on gut bacteria be responsible for this? It's still too soon to say for certain, but if you're watching your weight flaxseeds could be your ally.

MENOPAUSE

If you're a woman going through menopause, putting flaxseeds on the menu could also be a good move as several studies suggest that they may help ease menopausal symptoms. Again, in light of their high levels of lignans, which work like a low dose of oestrogen, this makes some sense. In one of the most intricate and ambitious studies, Turkish researchers compared the effects of flaxseeds with HRT on both menopausal symptoms and quality of life.

The women – 140 in all – were allocated to four groups. The first two were told to consume 5 grams of flaxseed a day and given tips on how to store and use them, while a third group took HRT, and a fourth received no treatment at all. In addition one of the flaxseed groups received training plus information on how to cope with menopause. All the women filled in symptom questionnaires and were asked about emotional problems, energy levels and fatigue, emotional well-being, social functioning, pain and general health to measure their quality of life.

At the end of three months both the HRT group and the flaxseed group saw a similar reduction in menopausal symptoms while, as you would expect, those who received no treatment whatsoever, saw an increase in menopausal symptoms. Better still, the women in both groups who consumed 5 grams of flaxseeds a day reported a greater improvement in their quality of life both compared with the HRT group or, again as you might expect, the no-treatment group. Bear in mind that, as mentioned above, any benefits could depend on your gut bacteria. But if you're going through menopause it might be worth adding a modest amount of flaxseeds to your diet – half a tablespoon a day, say – to see if they make a difference to how you feel.

INCONTINENCE

Without doubt, one of the most miserable and embarrassing mid-life problems is incontinence. So it's encouraging to learn that those lignans found in flaxseeds might just be able help with that too. At the time of writing there was no research specifically on flaxseeds, but in a study of 1,789 postmenopausal women aged 50+ from the Department of Urology, Massachusetts General Hospital, Boston, higher urine levels of one of the lignans found in flaxseeds was linked with a lower likelihood of incontinence. More studies are needed to discover exactly how lignans may have this effect, but if an irritable bladder or leaking is a problem, putting flaxseeds on the menu could be an easy way to boost those lignan levels.

BREAST CANCER

Lignans, together with that plant omega-3, ALA, found in flaxseeds, could also be behind the apparent potential of flaxseeds to help protect against breast cancer. Furthermore several studies from the lab bench suggest that ALA, may reduce the

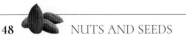

growth and size of breast cancer cells as well as putting a stop to their proliferation and even encouraging cancer cells to commit suicide. Lab experiments also show they can help boost the efficiency of the anti-breast cancer drug tamoxifen.

But what about outside the lab? Could putting flaxseeds on the menu help lower breast cancer risk in women? A decade or so ago, Canadian researchers reported findings from a study designed to answer this very question in women enrolled on one of the country's biggest studies of diet and health, the Ontario Women's Diet and Health Study. Their findings reported in the journal *Cancer Causes and Control* showed that both flaxseeds and flax bread were linked with a significant reduction in breast cancer risk. Now, as you're no doubt tired of reading just because two things are linked this doesn't prove that one causes the other, but it is an interesting finding, especially considering the results of other studies.

According to an article in the journal *Applied Physiology and Nutrient Metabolism* for example, clinical trials suggest that taking 25 grams of flaxseeds a day could reduce tumour growth in women with breast cancer. This fits in with other studies which have linked a higher intake of lignans (although not necessarily from flaxseeds) with a significant lowering of breast cancer in postmenopausal women according to a meta-analysis published in the *American Journal of Clinical Nutrition*.

A more recent study, which sought to find out how several different varieties of Egyptian flaxseeds might exert these potential anti-cancer effects, published in the journal *Clinical Reports*, meanwhile, showed that they caused cancer cells to commit suicide – something called apoptosis – as well as helping stall the growth of blood

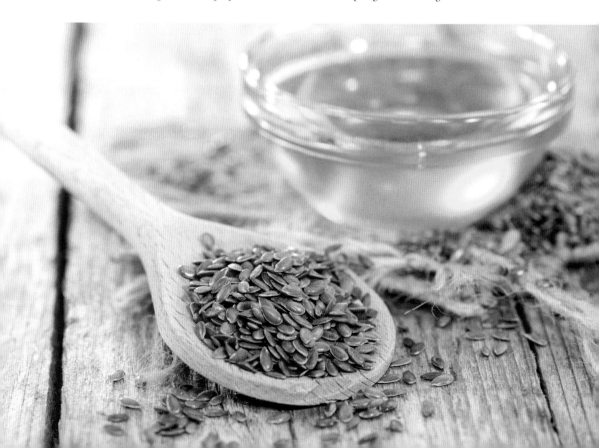

vessels serving tumours and stopping cancer cells from spreading. This study was only in mice so it's not possible to say whether the same effects would be seen in humans. But it does suggest one way in which flaxseeds could exert a potentially beneficial effect.

Clearly more studies – and especially more clinical trials in humans – are needed to find out exactly how many flaxseeds, in what form, when and for how long you need to consume them. Nevertheless the research is pointing in an interesting direction so keep an eye out for further studies.

Oh, one little tip if you're planning to add flaxseeds to your diet and you aren't used to eating a high fibre diet: take it slowly. Adding flaxseeds too quickly to your diet could upset your digestive system. And make sure you drink plenty of water too to encourage that fibre in flaxseeds to swell up and work as it should.

IN THE KITCHEN

Choose from whole seeds, flax oil and ground or milled flaxseed. Remember, grinding enables flaxseeds to be better digested and absorbed so maximising their nutrient benefits.

Add to breakfast cereals, meat and nut loaves, doughs, batters and cake or biscuit mixes

Stir into juices, smoothies and/or yoghurt and kefir.

Sprinkle sprouted flaxseeds over salads or use in homemade breads.

Mix ground flaxseeds into soups, stews and/or casseroles.

Add a spoonful of flaxseed oil to salad dressings to add flavour and nutrient value.

Use flaxseed water instead of egg in pancake, muffin, biscuit and cake mixes (one tbsp ground flaxseed with three tablespoons of water for one egg).

IT'S YOUR CHOICE...

To maximise lignans and other phytochemicals, let flaxseeds sprout for eight to ten days. Research has found that germinating flaxseeds for eight days boosts lignan levels around fivefold. Meanwhile the highest levels of those polyphenol and flavonoid plant chemicals appear to be found in 10-day germinated flaxseeds – with levels from six to fifty-five times more than in un-germinated seeds. The highest antioxidant and antiproliferative activities were also found on day ten.

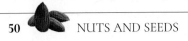

HAZELNUTS

Corylus avellana

According to research, these delicious, crunchy nuts with their hard glossy shells and sweet flavour could be your ally in helping to protect against heart disease and cancer and improve the health of the brain.

As well as being mentioned in Ancient Chinese texts 5,000 years ago, it's also clear from Greek and Roman writings that hazelnuts were cultivated in Europe too since classical times at least. These days they are most widely grown in Turkey, Italy, England and the US.

The second richest source among the tree nuts of heart-friendly MUFAs, mainly oleic acid, also found in olive oil, as well as plant sterols, vitamins and minerals including thiamin, vitamin B6, iron, and magnesium, alpha-tocopherol, a form of vitamin E, hazelnuts have pretty impressive credentials on the nutrition front. And that's even before taking into account their wealth of antioxidant phytochemicals, including proanthocyanidins found in apples, grapes, red wine and berries, and carotenoids found in red, yellow, orange and green veggies and fruit.

Hazelnuts, if you remember, are among the trio of nuts (the other two were walnuts and almonds) featured in the famous Spanish PREDIMED study of the benefits of a Mediterranean Diet, so their reputation goes before them. Clinical studies are fairly thin on the ground though, so what could they have got going for them?

HEART

Fast foods high in fat and refined carbs are key culprits in oxidative stress, a well-known factor in atherosclerosis, the furring and narrowing of the arteries, that can lead to heart attacks and strokes. So where better to test out the potential benefits of hazelnuts than McDonalds? That was the bright idea of Italian researchers who asked twenty-two volunteers to eat a McDonald's with a handful of hazelnuts.

Being Italian they didn't go for just any old hazelnuts, but chose Nocciole Tonda Gentile dell Langhe, a variety grown in the Piedmont area of Italy, much prized by gourmets who have voted them best in the world. Sure enough, consuming 40 grams of these hazelnuts helped quell oxidation of 'bad' LDL cholesterol, one of the key steps in hardening and narrowing of the arteries (atherosclerosis). How did they do this? Well the researchers also looked at 103 genes involved in inflammation and oxidative stress and found that hazelnuts blocked genes linked with inflammation and oxidative stress from being switched on.

But that may not be their only mechanism of action. With age our arteries become stiffer and less elastic and here's where hazelnuts look to score again. Another small Italian study, involving sixty-one healthy volunteers this time, found that consuming hazelnuts at breakfast boosted the elasticity of arteries as well as increasing levels of 'good' HDL cholesterol. And if you fancy a cup of cocoa (preferably without sugar) with your hazelnuts, go ahead. The study showed that cocoa and hazelnuts combined had even more benefits for arteries, yet another example of the synergy between foods.

Among the groups most at risk of heart disease are children and teenagers with high levels of blood fats. This is often due to a genetic condition called 'familial hyperlipidaemia', which puts them at risk of early heart disease. Italian researchers wanted to find out whether hazelnuts could protect against oxidative stress, DNA damage to cells caused by oxidation, the human equivalent of rusting.

In a study of sixty-six children reported in the *Journal of Nutritional Biochemistry*, it was found that just eight weeks of adding those much prized Tonda Gentile delle

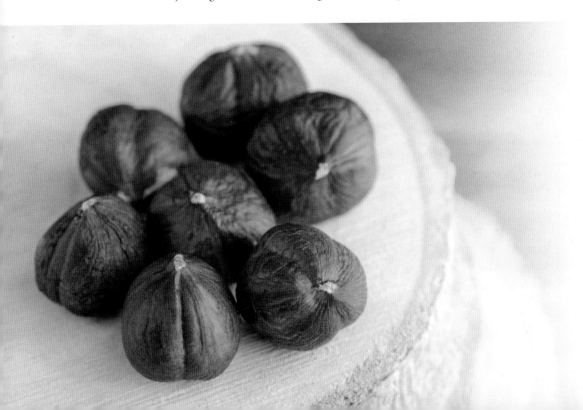

Langhe hazelnuts to the diet almost halved tell-tale signs of DNA damage, a finding that mirrors studies in adults who supplemented their diets with other nuts including almonds or Brazil nuts or mixed nuts (walnuts, almonds and hazelnuts).

These are all pretty small, preliminary studies and many of them seem like an advert for Tonda Gentile delle Langhe. Nevertheless they do give a hint of how hazelnuts may help protect against heart disease as well as adding to the considerable evidence showing that a Mediterranean diet including nuts can help reduce the risk of cardiovascular problems.

BRAIN

In Persian Traditional Medicine, hazelnuts have long been said to help prevent the brain shrinkage – aka cerebral atrophy – that accompanies dementia caused by Alzheimer's disease (AD). So could there be any truth in this? In an attempt to find out, Iranian scientists looked at the effects of hazelnuts on Alzheimer's disease. Their findings, published in *Nutritional Neuroscience*, showed that adding hazelnuts to the diet boosted memory and reduced anxiety-related behaviour. But again there's that caveat: in lab animals. They also helped quell neuroinflammation and cell death caused by beta-amyloid, the main component of the hallmark 'plaques' found in the brains of people with Alzheimer's disease. The researchers suggest that supplementing the diet with hazelnuts could boost healthy ageing and benefit people with Alzheimer's.

Another Iranian study of hazelnuts, almonds and walnuts published in the journal *Pharmacological Research* provides some hints as to why this might be. It found that nutrients and plant chemicals found in hazelnuts targeted underlying mechanisms involved in AD such as the protein 'plaques and tangles' found in the brains of people with the disease, as well as helping to combat oxidative stress, caused by free radical attack and other factors such as lowering cholesterol and inflammation and the formation of new brain cells (neurogenesis).

Although these findings have come from lab tests, and animals not people, they do fit in with a growing number of studies showing that nuts may benefit brain health. The long-running US Nurses' Health Study found that women who consume larger amounts of nuts have better cognition in later life. You've read it before but once again it seems to be a matter of: watch this space.

CANCER

Studies of the positive benefits of hazelnuts have so far mainly focused on heart health. But research is emerging that they could also have a role in helping to protect against cancer. For example, although not specific to hazelnuts, one study reported at the 2017 meeting of the American Society of Clinical Oncology revealed that bowel cancer patients who consumed two or more ounces of nuts (including hazelnuts and other tree nuts) a week – around one in five participants – had a 42 per cent lower risk of their cancer returning and a 57 per cent lower risk of dying than non-nut eaters. The study included 826 patients being treated for stage 3 colon cancer meaning that their cancer had begun to spread to nearby lymph nodes. What studies like this can't tell us, of course, is whether the nuts account for this, or whether other factors – for example generally healthier eating habits or lifestyle – are responsible.

To try and tease out the specific effects of hazelnuts we have to turn back to the lab, where an interesting piece of research published in the journal *Anticancer Research* showed that hazelnuts – both raw and roasted – had the ability to block the growth of colon cancer cells, in a test tube. Meanwhile in yet another study published in *Food Chemistry*, hamsters that were fed a high-fat diet and were given extracts of hazelnut skin had a lower level of two 'bile acids' produced by the gallbladder, which have been linked with an increased risk of both bowel cancer and heart disease.

A couple of studies don't prove anything very much of course, especially when they have come out of the lab rather than being done on humans. But they certainly lend weight to the suggestion that a diet rich in nuts could help protect against cancer. And what we do know is that hazelnut skins are exceptionally rich in some of those antioxidant, anti-inflammatory polyphenols as well as having a high percentage of fibre, which gets fermented in the gut to produce compounds called short-chain fatty

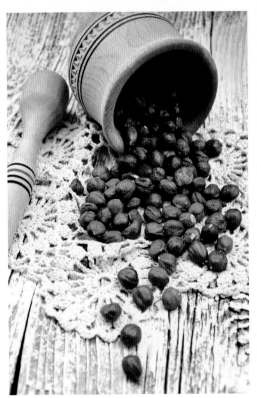

acids (SCFA) that are thought, among other things, to help deter the formation of cancer cells. Could this help explain their potential anticancer effects? It's certainly a possibility, and one that is a good reason for making hazelnuts part of your diet.

DID YOU KNOW?

It's not just the nuts of the hazel tree that may have benefits. Scientists have discovered that paclitaxel, a powerful anti-cancer compound extracted from the bark of yew trees which is the basis for the anticancer drug Taxol® is to be found in the stems, leaves and shells of hazelnuts. This tantalising finding could pave the way to the use of paclitaxel from hazelnut 'waste' being used in anti-cancer medications.

IN THE KITCHEN

Pound with polyphenol-rich roasted red-pepper and grilled tomatoes, ground almonds, olive oil and red vinegar to make the famous Catalan salsa romesco – great spread on a slice of sourdough toast.

Mix with a Mediterranean herb such as oregano and mascarpone, ricotta or cream and for a quick mild pasta sauce – add chilli and wilted spinach, or bitter greens if you can get hold of them, for a spicier more complex variation.

Combine with anchovies, garlic and olive oil and whizz up for a different take on pesto – serve with asparagus spears or sprouting broccoli stalks.

Mix with breadcrumbs and use as a healthy crispy coating for fried or baked fish fillets.

Brown in butter or oil and use as a topping for fish and seafood dishes such as cod, halibut or scallops.

Roast or toast, chop roughly and use to top summer salads or lasagne.

Add to roasted cauliflower, eggs, cream and thyme for a veggie take on pasta carbonara,

Drizzle hazelnut oil over salads.

Spread hazelnut butter over your morning toast or crispbread for a mid-morning or afternoon snack

Add crunch to savoury quiches and tarts – they have an especial affinity for mushrooms (try mixed mushrooms for an extra dose of polyphenols).

Chop and add to fried onions and breadcrumbs in stuffings or stuffing balls – they combine especially well with dried apricots.

Add chopped to Indian pilaus, risottos, biryanis and other rice dishes.

Top hearty winter soups such a Brussels sprouts, leek and potato or celeriac soup with toasted chopped hazelnuts and a swirl of oil.

Stir into yoghurt for a quick dessert or add to smoothies for a breakfast treat.

Use in baking – biscuits, such as the Italian biscotti, cakes, meringues and cheesecakes all benefit from the addition of chopped hazelnuts. Alternatively if you can get hold of it or make your own, use hazelnut paste instead of almond marzipan.

IT'S YOUR CHOICE...

Don't rub off the skins! Many recipes suggest rubbing off hazelnut skins. However as many of the beneficial antioxidant plant compounds and of course fibre thought to be responsible for their health benefits reside in their skin this may not be so clever. Prefer your nuts dry roasted and lightly salted? Go ahead and enjoy; this does not affect their potential benefits, and a Turkish study published in the journal, *Food Chemistry,* found roasted hazelnut skins to be especially high in heart-friendly phytonutrients.

HEMP SEEDS

Cannabis Sativa L.

Hemp seeds are widely available as whole hulled seeds (aka hemp nuts or hemp hearts), as a delicious nutty oil and in the plant protein powders that are becoming increasingly popular. Scientists are at last beginning to look at the potential health benefits which, it seems, could be significant.

An important food, fibre and medicine since prehistoric times, hemp's medicinal properties feature in Egyptian papyruses. In modern times, however, at least until pretty recently, hemp – and its derivatives – have suffered from their association with their more infamous relative, marijuana. And it's perhaps this damning reputation that also accounts for the surprising scarcity of research on their effects on the body.

So let's get this straight: the seeds of the industrial hemp plant from which food hemp seeds derive have exceptionally low levels of tetrahydrocannabinoids (THC), the active ingredient in marijuana, meaning that consuming them won't make you high. And that's potentially good news because hemp seeds' star seems to be on the ascendant.

Oh, just one more thing before we get on to the real nitty gritty: hemp-seed oil is different from cannabidiol oil or CBD which is causing a big noise at the moment and which is extracted from the leaves and flowers of industrial hemp.

Hemp seeds are exceptionally rich in plant proteins – they contain almost as much protein as soya beans – including high levels of the amino acid, arginine, which is thought to contribute to the health of the arteries. They also contain vitamins and minerals including vitamin E, phosphorus, potassium, sodium, magnesium, sulphur, calcium, iron and zinc, as well as an unusual mixture of fats and fatty acids, many of which have proven health benefits. Last but not least they contain a variety of phytonutrients some of which are unique to hemp. Let's take a peek at some of those potential health benefits in more detail.

HEART

The presence of omega-6 and omega-3 PUFAs in hemp seeds and the amino acid, arginine, which is changed into nitric acid in the body, which is thought to have benefits for the elasticity of the arteries, suggests that both hemp seeds and their oil could, in theory at least, benefit heart health. And sure enough, in animals they have been found to have strong blood-pressure lowering, cholesterol-lowering and anti-clotting effects, so there could be something to this.

Hemp seeds have also been found to help protect against damage to heart tissue which happens when the heart is deprived of oxygen during a heart attack and blood flow is restored too fast, something doctors call ischemia-reperfusion injury, or IRI.

In a study by scientists from the Canadian Centre for Agri-food Research in Health and Medicine rats were put on a diet supplemented with hemp seeds. Other rats were fed a diet enriched with palm oil, which is high in saturated fats, and others with partially defatted hempseeds for twelve weeks.

After a period of oxygen deprivation tests were carried out on their hearts. And guess what? The hearts of the rats fed on hemp seed recovered significantly better than those fed on palm oil, suggesting that hemp seeds could help protect against IRI.

So far, so promising. But of course, as so often, it's a far cry from animals to people, a point underlined in one of the few human studies on hemp-seed oil for the heart. This compared the effects of taking two one gram capsules of hemp seed oil, fish oil, flax-seed oil or a dummy capsule every day for twelve weeks on risk factors for heart disease including blood fats, inflammation and clotting in eighty-six healthy men and women. Disappointingly there were no effects.

It could be, of course, that this study did not go on long enough, or perhaps the dose was not high enough or there was some other reason. And indeed a subsequent small, randomised, controlled trial published in the *European Journal of Nutrition* found that taking 30 millilitres of hemp oil led to a lower total cholesterol-to-HDL cholesterol ratio compared with flax-seed oil, something that has been linked to a lower risk of heart disease. However this was only a small study – just fourteen people in all – and other studies looking at the effects of hemp-seed oil on blood fats other aspects of heart disease have been inconclusive.

Clearly there are still gaps in our knowledge about hemp seed and in particular, according to a review published in the journal *Nutrition and Metabolism*, we need more

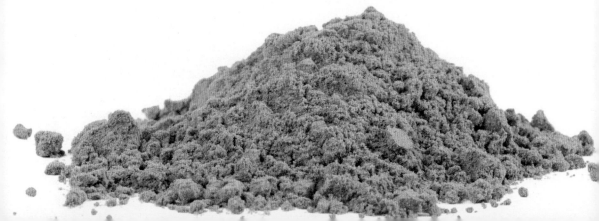

information about how bioavailable (how easily absorbed and used) the fatty acids in hemp seeds are, and whether the age or sex of the person, or indeed the hemp seed, itself plays a part in this.

PROTEIN POWER

That's where matters seemed to rest until recently, but it's not just the fats in hemp seeds that are now attracting attention. In the past few years researchers have begun to examine the potential benefits of hemp-seed protein, and these are showing promise.

For example, if you're diagnosed with high cholesterol or high blood pressure, the doctor may recommend first taking steps to change your diet and lifestyle before prescribing medication. And consuming fewer animal and more plant-based foods is often one of those recommendations. So the news that small protein fragments, or peptides, found in hemp-seed protein powder could help lower both cholesterol and blood pressure is welcome.

In fact, according to an Italian study published in the *Journal of Agricultural and Food chemistry*, it seems that hemp-seed protein could even act like medication. This found that extracts of hemp-seed protein acted like statins. Another study published in the same journal found that hemp-seed peptides worked in a way similar to ACE-inhibitors, drugs commonly used to lower blood pressure.

Both these studies were on cells in a test tube – and of course, as always, it's important to bear in mind that test-tube research can only tell us so much. Nevertheless, it's an intriguing finding and one that might prompt you to consider adding hemp protein powder to your morning smoothie.

INFLAMMATION

Inflammation, as you know, is now thought to be a contributory factor to a host of diseases. And the fatty acid profile of hemp seeds is such that it could, in principle, have a role to play in helping to combat this. The reason? Hemp seeds are rich in another PUFA, gamma linolenic acid (GLA), which may be familiar as the main fatty acid in evening primrose and borage oils. They also contain another omega-3 fatty acid, stearidonic acid, also found in blackcurrants. And it turns out that both of these can block inflammation.

ECZEMA

In light of this it's interesting to discover that in one of the few studies on eczema sufferers who took two tablespoons (30 millilitres) of cold-pressed hemp-seed oil experienced a significant improvement in dryness and itching and were able to reduce topical medication in just eight weeks. The researchers, whose paper was published in the *Journal of Dermatological Treatment*, attribute this to 'the balanced and abundant supply of PUFAs in this hempseed oil'. Just one small study, true, but one that seems to be pointing the right way.

RHEUMATOID ARTHRITIS

What about other inflammatory diseases? Well, hemp seeds have been used for centuries in traditional Korean and Chinese medicine to treat rheumatoid arthritis (RA), a debilitating, chronic disease of the joints. RA can be difficult to treat, not least because cells lining the joints, which produce inflammatory chemicals, refuse to die and instead fight back against one of the most common treatments. Much research in RA is now focused on these cells and how to kill them. So a lab-based Korean study which found that adding hempseed oil to these cells in a test tube caused them to commit suicide is encouraging. But again this is just in the lab and there are no studies in humans.

CONSTIPATION

In traditional Chinese medicine, hemp seeds have long been used as a laxative. But is there any science behind this? A randomised, controlled trial of ninety-six people with chronic constipation by the Hong Kong Baptist University published in the *American Journal of Gastroenterology*, found that eight weeks of taking Chinese hemp-seed pills helped restore bowel function and ease constipation and straining. The optimum dose? In this study 7.5 grams.

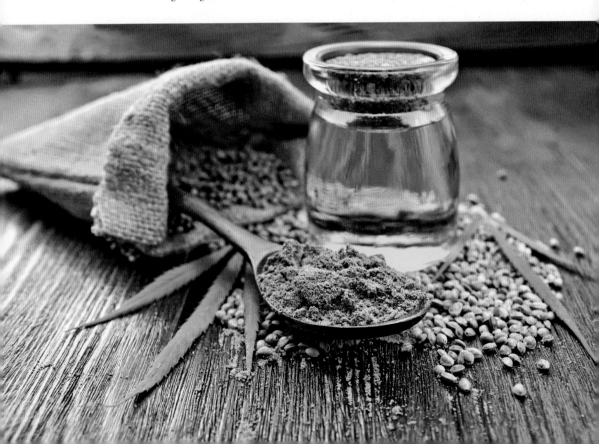

The take-home message? It is clear that there's still a huge amount we need to learn about hemp seeds. Having said that, the wealth of nutrients they contain means that they could be a valuable addition to your diet. And who knows they could even help you to better health?

IN THE KITCHEN

Top cereals, salads and yogurts with hulled hemp seeds for an extra protein boost.

Stir hemp seed protein powder into to porridge, overnight oats, smoothies or shakes.

If you're avoiding gluten use hemp seeds instead of breadcrumbs to coat fish or chicken before frying.

Swirl hemp-seed oil over soups and salads or use to top pasta or oven bakes – don't heat it up though or you will destroy those valuable oils.

IT'S YOUR CHOICE...

Seek out the cold-pressed hemp-seed oil. Cold pressing helps to preserve nutrients including gamma-tocopherol, a kind of vitamin E which protects the oil from oxidation both in the bottle and the body

MACADAMIAS

Macadamia integrifolia/tetraphylla

A lthough not as well researched as other tree nuts and given only a cautious thumbs up from the experts until fairly recently, macadamia nuts are currently rising up the nutrition charts for their potential ability to help heart health, quell inflammation and even possibly help manage weight.

Native to Australia, where they are sometimes known as Queensland nuts, macadamias were a well-kept secret of the Aboriginal peoples, for whom gathering the nuts they called kindal kindal, boombera, jindill or baupal was an autumn ritual for millennia. Until 1858 that is, when a German-Australian botanist, Ferdinand von Mueller, stumbled across the evergreen tree with its shiny, dark-green leaves and named it macadamia after his friend and colleague, Dr John Macadam. And so was born an industry which, in today's Australia, encompasses 700 macadamia farmers

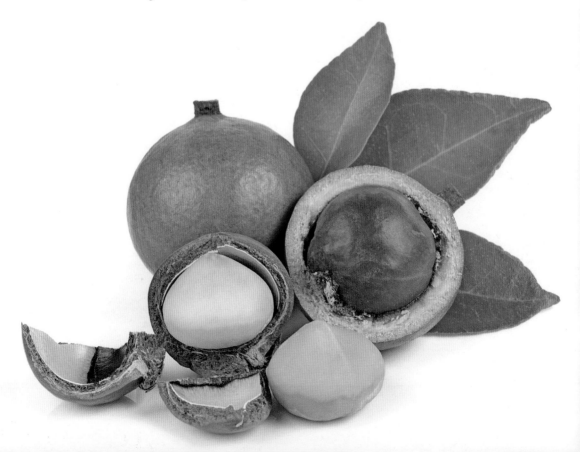

growing 6.9 million trees covering 22,000 hectares of land, mainly in Queensland and New South Wales. Macadamia nuts are also important crops in South Africa, Hawaii, Kenya and Brazil.

With their soft, creamy texture, rich, sweetish taste and irresistible crunch, it's easy to see why macadamia nuts are such a popular snack. And as a source of carbohydrates, fibre, protein together with a variety of vitamins and minerals including B vitamins, calcium, iron, magnesium, phosphorus, potassium and plant chemicals and an unusually high MUFA content they are fast gaining a reputation for their health benefits too. So what are these?

HEART

Gram for gram there's no doubt macadamias are one of the fattiest nuts. It's what gives them that moreish crunch and rich, buttery flavour. It was this high fat content, that gained them such a bad rap among dietitians and nutritionists until relatively recently. But what the experts who told us not to eat too many macadamias failed to take into account, was that the main fats in macadamia nuts are those MUFAs which are linked with a more heart friendly blood fat profile.

So could eating macadamia nuts benefit heart health? That's the question Hawaiian researchers set out to answer in a study reported in the journal *Archives of Internal Medicine* back in 2000. They compared blood fat levels of thirty healthy volunteers who first ate a 'typical American diet', then the low-fat diet at that time recommended by the American Heart Association (AHA), and subsequently a diet which included macadamia nuts.

Their findings? Not only did the macadamia-supplemented diet lower total and 'bad' LDL cholesterol to the same extent as the low-fat AHA diet, it also lowered levels of other blood fats called triglycerides, which are linked with a higher risk of heart disease and type 2 diabetes.

Now the people in this study were all healthy with normal cholesterol levels. The question is could macadamias help those with high cholesterol? Another study published in the *Journal of Nutrition*, this time of seventeen men with high cholesterol levels, suggests they could. It found that adding macadamia nuts to their diets resulted in total and 'bad' LDL cholesterol levels going down and 'good' HDL cholesterol levels rising. Two small studies only, but there could be something in them.

MUFA MAGIC

What accounts these apparently favourable effects on cholesterol? Well for a start macadamia nuts have the highest ratio of MUFAs to PUFAs (polyunsaturated fatty acids) of all tree nuts, something that many experts consider desirable when it comes to blood fat health. What's more, the main MUFA in macadamias is oleic acid,

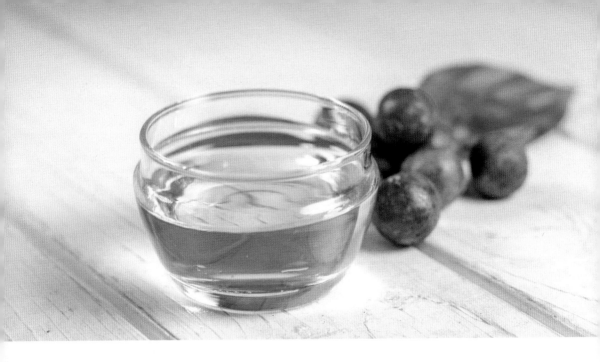

also found in olive oil, widely considered to be one of the secrets of the Mediterranean diet when it comes to matters of the heart.

What's perhaps less well known, except among nutrition experts, is that macadamia nuts are also abundant in another MUFA that goes by the name of palmitoleic acid. This is an omega-7 fatty acid also found in salmon, in the shrub sea buckthorn, chocolate, olive oil and eggs. The jury is still out on its effects, but there is some research suggesting that it could help reduce the incidence of type 2 diabetes as well as having a favourable effect on blood fats. The evidence is still fairly unclear and at times downright contradictory, but it's worth keeping an eye out for developments.

INSULIN RESISTANCE AND WEIGHT

Heart disease, as you may have realised if you've read other entries, is pretty far down the line of a long trail of disturbances in body chemistry that starts with being overweight, especially fat around the middle, and insulin resistance, when the body can't use insulin properly. So, if you'll forgive the pun, it's heartening to learn that in lab studies at least, macadamia nuts, macadamia oil and palmitoleic acid seem capable of improving these. But what about in humans? Again it has to be admitted that there is, as yet, no very clear picture.

On the one hand some, although not all, studies show that palmitoleic acid can help protect against these. What's more, palmitoleic acid also seems to show promise in reducing inflammation, something we know is involved in the development of heart disease and diabetes as well as other chronic diseases. On the other hand there still aren't yet enough really convincing studies in humans. As so often, it's a matter of watching and waiting until the research is more conclusive.

NUTS AND SEEDS

WEIGHT

Could macadamias – or the MUFAs they contain – help manage weight? The findings of a small Japanese study published in the journal *Clinical and Experimental Pharmacology and Physiology* offer this as a tantalising possibility, as does another study originally designed to test the effects of macadamias on cholesterol levels.

In this, study seventy-one healthy women students all aged around 19 years were invited to add two loaves of bread fortified with either 10 grams of macadamia nuts, or the same amount of coconut or butter to their diet.

As in the studies already outlined, the women eating the macadamia-fortified bread had lower levels both of total and 'bad' LDL cholesterol, especially compared with the group eating butter. No surprise there then. What's more intriguing, though, is that both their body weight and BMI were significantly lower than those who ate the butter or coconut breads.

As so often, this study is simply too small to allow us to draw any firm conclusions on whether macadamias – or the MUFAs they contain – can help control weight. However, it does suggest that even if you're watching your weight you don't have to strike macadamias from your diet.

So what's the verdict on macadamias? Well, the American Academy of Nutrition and Dietetics deemed the evidence on them sufficient to advise a diet that 'includes the regular consumption of a variety of nuts (including macadamia nuts)' as part of its dietary recommendations. However as yet the studies of macadamias specifically are all over the place, so unfortunately it's not really possible to draw any firm conclusions. However, if macadamia nuts are your thing, as long as you don't go overboard, it looks as if you can grab yourself a handful now and then with a clear conscience.

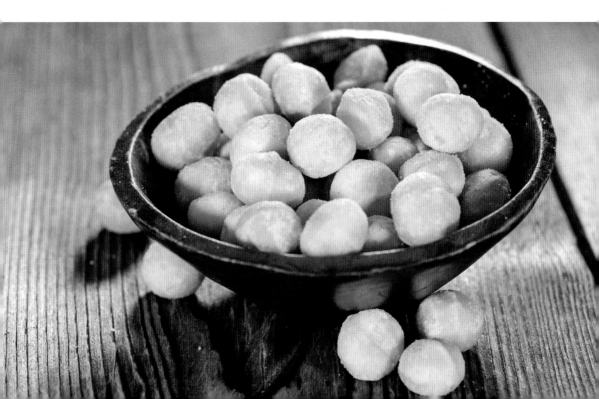

IN THE KITCHEN

Snack on a handful of raw macadamia nuts or add them other nuts and trail mixes.

Add whole to salads for a nutritious crunch.

Chop and add to bread or nut loaves or rissoles.

Add to smoothies.

Use to top yogurt and breakfast bowls.

Roasted with spices of your choice plus a squeeze of lime or lemon and a drizzle of honey they make a great snack to hand round with drinks.

Add to bakes, cakes and biscuits for an occasional treat.

Use macadamia nut oil in salad dressings.

Alternatively apply it to your skin for a beauty boost – it's said to have a chemical profile similar to the natural oils produced by the skin.

IT'S YOUR CHOICE...

Like your macadamias roasted – and who doesn't? If you're doing it yourself you'll get the best quality by roasting at 115°C (240°F) for 19–35 min, 125°C (257°F) for 10–14 min or 135°C (275°F) for 4 min, so says research in the *Journal of the Science of Food and Agriculture*.

PEANUTS

Arachis hypogaea

And so to peanuts, not just just the most popular nuts in the world, but ironically not even nuts. Exceptionally high in nutrients they contain all the amino acids we need for health as well as being a source of folate, vitamin E, the minerals magnesium, manganese, and phosphorus together with those heart and brain-friendly MUFAs (monounsaturated fatty acids).

In recent years peanuts, especially their skins, have been recognised as a source par excellence of a whole range of phytochemicals and plant sterols that block absorption of cholesterol. Peanuts are also a source of co-enzyme Q10, which our cells need for energy production. In other words they are pretty packed with healthy nutrients.

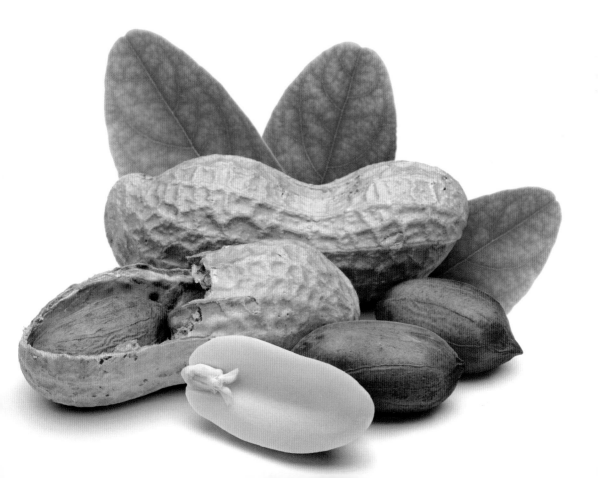

What you may be surprised to hear, however, is that peanuts are actually legumes – plants whose fruits or seeds come in a shell or pod – meaning they are more closely related to peas, beans and lentils than to almonds, walnuts, hazelnuts and the rest of the tree nuts.

Whatever their provenance, it seems we humans have always been crazy for them. In 2007 US anthropologists discovered wild peanut remains in sealed house floors and hearths, beneath grinding stones and in stone-lined storage units buried in a tropical dry forest of the Ñanchoc Valley on the lower western slopes of the Andes in north Peru. This find provides the first evidence of our hunter-gatherer ancestors liking for peanuts some 8,000 years ago.

And still today our appetite for peanuts seems unstoppable. Depending where in the world you live you'll find them whole, plain, roasted, as that favourite toast topper, peanut butter, as well as in peanut (groundnut) oil, peanut sauce, peanut 'milk', and peanut snack bars. In fact so popular are they that we get through two-and-a-half times more peanuts than all other nuts combined. They are also widely used in the food industry in peanut flour and oil.

Good news on the health front as in recent years they have gone from being persona non grata on account of their high fat content to being hailed as a functional food. So what have they got going for them?

HEART

As so often, the most compelling research relates to the potential benefits of peanuts for the heart. Peanuts are among the nuts studied in three of the best regarded, long-running health studies: the Nurses' Health Study, which ran from 1980–2012 and included 76,364 women; the Nurses' Health Study 2, which ran from 1991–2013 and included 92,946 women; and the Health Professionals Follow-up Study, which ran from 1986–2012 and included 41,526 male health professionals.

In a review by Harvard scientists looking at the links between nut consumption and the risk of heart disease, consuming peanuts and tree nuts twice or more a week was linked with a 13–19 per cent lower risk of all types of heart disease and 15–23per cent lower risk of CHD – aka coronary heart disease – caused by furring and narrowing of the arteries.

And these promising findings, published in the *Journal of the American College of Cardiology*, are echoed in studies of people of different ethnicity, leading the authors of another review, this time published in *Progress in Cardiovascular Disease*, to suggest that overall 'observational studies' – ones that look for links between certain foods and particular health outcomes – show a consistent heart protective effect for peanuts. This applies across the spectrum from non-fatal heart attack to fatal heart attack, sudden cardiac death in men and women of different ages, background and areas of the world. Praise indeed for peanuts.

Of course, as you're aware by now, correlation doesn't equal cause and effect, so what about the possible effects of peanuts specifically on those blood fats? A US study of fifteen people with a normal blood fat profile who substituted part of their diet with peanuts or other fats for three weeks, or an equal amount of other fats for eight weeks, found that peanuts resulted in lower levels of triglycerides, blood fats that are linked with a higher risk of heart disease and type 2 diabetes.

The addition of peanuts also increased levels of dietary fibre, magnesium, folate, vitamin E, copper all of which are linked to a reduced risk of heart disease as well as the amino acid, arginine, which is thought to help improve the elasticity of the arteries. Although admittedly small, this study published in the *Journal of the American College of Nutrition* does provide a rationale for the effects of peanuts on health, and supports other studies that have shown that a high nut intake is linked to a lower risk of heart disease.

BRAIN

You'll be familiar by now with the idea that what is good for the heart is good for the brain, although there have been few studies specifically on peanuts for brain health. Nevertheless if you are thinking of going nuts for peanuts there's one variety you may want to consider choosing for the sake of that grey matter. Called high oleic peanuts, they are available as kernels or in peanut butter. And the reason why you may want to have a pack in your kitchen cupboard is that they are especially high in the heart-friendly MUFA, oleic acid, the main fat in olive oil, thought to be partly responsible for the health benefits of a Mediterranean diet, as well as of plant sterols.

In a trial by Australian researchers, sixty-one healthy, but overweight, men and women were asked to consume their normal diet first for twelve weeks and then to supplement this with 56–84 grams a day of high-oleic peanuts. At the end of the study, published in *Nutritional Neuroscience*, the researchers measured the health of blood vessels serving their brains. And you know what? After consuming the high oleic peanuts their small arteries were 10 per cent more elastic. The researchers also assessed their cognitive function and found that their short-term memory, verbal fluency and processing speed (the speed at which the brain processes information) were higher. An encouraging result if you're a peanut lover.

WEIGHT

And those high oleic peanuts could also have another benefit. It seems they are less likely to pile on the kilos – perhaps as a result of their high MUFA content than regular peanuts. Research published in the journal *Obesity* has shown that high oleic peanuts can help reduce inflammation and help balance blood glucose levels in overweight/obese men. Meanwhile a Brazilian study, published in the journal

Nutricia Hospitalaria, researchers found that a group of overweight and obese men who substituted high oleic peanuts for ordinary peanuts burned a greater number of calories after eating, as well as feeling fuller. All of which suggests they could be a good choice of snack if you're trying to cut back on less healthy snacks such as crisps, biscuits, cakes or sweets.

Looking for another reason to pick high oleic peanuts? Their high MUFA content means they are less susceptible to going rancid than regular peanuts and so have a longer shelf life, something worth bearing in mind next time you go to pick a pack off the supermarket shelf.

DIABETES

Several studies suggest that nuts – including peanuts – may help protect against type 2 diabetes, so the results of the famous US Nurses' Health Study are interesting. The Nurses' Health Study is, in the words of Donna Shalala, the former Secretary of the US Department of Health and Human Services, 'one of the most significant studies ever conducted on the health of women'. So when findings are published people sit up and take notice.

In 1980 researchers from the study began tracking the health of 83,818 women aged 34–59 years from eleven US states. All were free of diabetes, cardiovascular disease, or cancer at the start of the study. The women were asked to fill in a food questionnaire and were tracked for sixteen years. At the end of this time 3,206 of them had

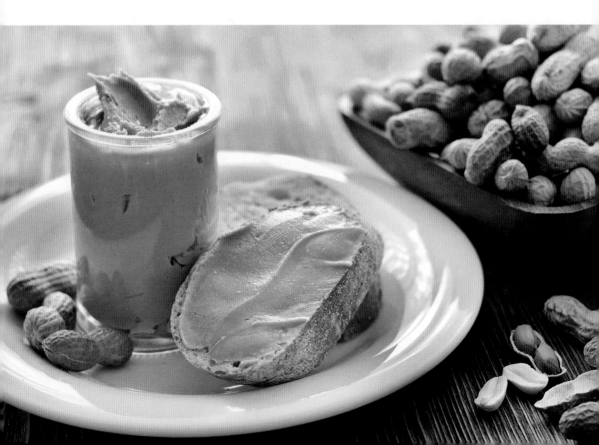

developed type 2 diabetes. The researchers discovered that those women who ate the most nuts – including peanuts – were the least likely to develop diabetes – a finding that still held true even after allowing for BMI, smoking, alcohol consumption, and other diabetes risk factors.

And, here's some potential good news. if you're a peanut-butter-on-toast fan, they also found that women who ate peanut butter five times or more a week (equivalent to 140 grams or around 5 oz of peanuts a week) were 11 per cent less likely to develop type 2 diabetes than study participants who rarely ate peanut butter. Of course, as you're no doubt sick of reading by now, just because two things are linked it doesn't prove that one causes the other, and it could just reflect the fact the peanut butter lovers eat a healthier diet generally but it's certainly an interesting result if you prefer your peanuts as a spread rather than in a packet.

CANCER

As with other nuts, most research on peanuts has tended to focus on their effects on heart disease and diabetes. But could they also help protect against cancer? Some tantalising hints are emerging. A study in *Cancer Causes and Control* from scientists at Maastricht University, for example, found a link between peanut consumption – although not peanut butter – and a lower risk of a type of breast cancer, called ER negative breast cancer in post-menopausal women.

This echoes the results of an earlier Italian study, which found that a high consumption of peanuts (as well as walnuts or almonds) was linked to a two or threefold lower risk of breast cancer. Other research published in the *World Journal of Gastroenterology* found that women who ate higher amounts of peanuts had a lower risk of bowel cancer.

It has to be admitted that this research is really still at too early a stage to draw any firm conclusions but it's certainly plausible that peanuts – especially if you leave their skins on – could be part of an anti-cancer arsenal. The reason? They are a source of one of the most researched polyphenols, resveratrol, also found in grape skins and red wine. Studies suggest resveratrol may encourage the suicide of cancer cells, medically called apoptosis, as well as helping prevent cancer cells from invading surrounding tissue, blocking the formation of blood vessels which tumours need to fuel their growth, helping control on-off switches in genes linked with cancer and interfering with chemical pathways that may lead to cancer.

MENTAL HEALTH

Talking of resveratrol, recent research suggests that it could have a role to play in mental health. In recent years experts have been investigating the role that brain inflammation might play in depression and have discovered that stress and depression are linked with increased production of inflammatory chemicals by

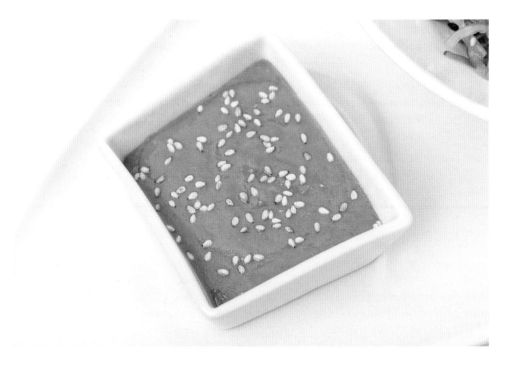

the immune system. They have also discovered that oxidative stress – the human equivalent of rusting remember – is involved in depression and the more oxidative stress there is, the more severe and long lasting the depression.

In a review published in *Molecular Neurobiology*, US and Brazilian researchers suggest that the proven antioxidant and anti-inflammatory properties of resveratrol could have beneficial effects for the brain citing studies showing that it supresses brain inflammation and may help improve learning, memory, anxiety, and depression at least in experimental studies in cells and animals. There are, as yet, virtually no studies of resveratrol as a treatment for depression in humans – and none whatsoever on whether peanuts might improve mood. It's a fascinating area of study however, so although it's a far stretch to recommend peanuts for mood once again, it's a matter of 'watch this space'.

IN THE KITCHEN

Snack on roasted or dry roasted peanuts.

Add a handful of roast peanuts to salads and stir fries – they have a particular affinity for Asian flavours such as that classic combination of sesame oil, chillies, spring onions, fish sauce, lime and coriander leaves.

Grind your own peanuts or cheat and use peanut butter in West African inspired soups and stews – you'll find lots of recipes online.

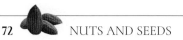

Toss into Indian curries or add to steamed or fried rice to accompany these.

Roast and grind and add to South Indian style groundnut chutney – again look for recipes online.

Make peanut sauce to accompany fish, chicken or tofu kebabs or serve with salads or drizzle over steamed veggies such as broccoli or asparagus.

Use non-salted peanuts in sweet dishes such as bakes, cakes, biscuits and deserts.

Use unrefined – and preferably cold-pressed – peanut oil in salad dressings, or drizzle over vegetables for a change from olive oil.

Fry with refined peanut oil – its bland flavour and high smoking point also make it great for frying.

IT'S YOUR CHOICE...

To enhance the antioxidant powers of peanuts, add to stews or other dishes that involve boiling. Research has found that boiling peanuts increases levels of antioxidant plant chemicals called isoflavones two- to four-fold. This applies to raw peanuts of course, *not* the roasted, salted kind.

PECAN NUTS

Carya illinoinensis

C ontaining an abundance of healthy fats, fibre and other nutrients, this relative of the walnut with its crinkled shape, reddish-brown skin, creamy texture and sweetish taste could have significant benefits for the health of your heart and brain.

Long before Columbus set sail for the Americas, pecans, the fruit of a species of hickory tree, was an important part in the diet of indigenous tribes living in central and southern areas of what is now the USA. Today they are best known for their starring role on the Thanksgiving dinner table. But, as you will discover, there is more to pecans than pecan pie.

Sharing second place with walnuts as the world's most popular nut, gram for gram pecans are also the fattiest. Fully half of their nutrient content is fat. Most of which consists of MUFAs and in particular oleic acid, the main fatty acid in olive oil, and PUFAs linked with a healthier blood fat profile.

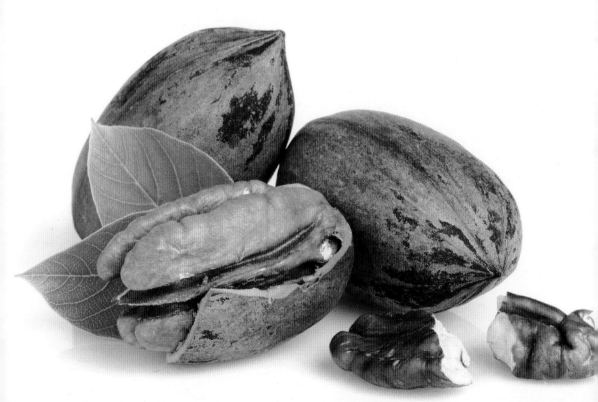

They also contain a plant form of that plant omega-3 PUFA, ALA, aka alpha-linolenic acid as well as plant sterols, naturally occurring compounds that help reduce cholesterol together with other biologically active plant chemicals, which help to usher fats in and out of our body's cells.

But these aren't the only things pecans have going for them. They also contain fibre, vitamin E, essential minerals including magnesium, manganese and zinc plus a wealth of polyphenols. Think, specifically, proanthocyanidins, also found in grapes, apples, berries, gallic and ellagic acid, also found in pomegranate juice, and a variety of flavonoids, such as catechins and gallocatechins, found in green tea – all of which have been linked with health benefits. So which areas of health might they benefit? Let's take a look.

HEART DISEASE AND DIABETES

You may have read that pecans can help combat heart problems. But they haven't attracted nearly as much specific research as other tree nuts. Nevertheless, a number of studies have looked at how pecans affect cholesterol and other harmful blood fats which are linked with a higher risk of heart disease.

One of the earliest pieces of research was a small US study, published in the *Journal of the American Dietary Association*, in which researchers asked five men and eighteen women all with healthy cholesterol levels to consume 68 grams of pecan halves a day or to avoid nuts altogether. Other than this they were allowed to eat whatever they chose. At the end of eight weeks, the researchers measured their blood fats and found that those who had added pecans to their diet had significantly lower levels of both 'bad' LDL and total cholesterol. A small study, but suggestive.

Another small US study following shortly afterwards reported in the *Journal of Nutrition* went a step further. It found that people who added pecans to their diet had lower LDL cholesterol and other blood fats called triglycerides, as well as higher levels of 'good' HDL cholesterol, than a matched group who consumed the low-fat heart-healthy diet recommended at that time by the American Heart Association.

What was especially interesting about this study is that the pecan-enriched diet contained quite a bit more fat (around 40 grams compared to 28 grams) than the heart-healthy diet. Of course these days researchers argue that when it comes to heart health, it's the kinds of fat we consume that we need to be most aware of. But back then, when we were all being advised to avoid consuming too many nuts on the grounds they were too fatty, this must have come as something of a revelation.

What is it in pecans that makes them so potentially beneficial to the blood fat profile? Well, you already know about their abundance of MUFAs and PUFAs, and in a study reported in the *Journal of Nutrition*, researchers at Loma Linda University in California added another piece to the emerging jigsaw. Pecans are rich in several nutrients including a form of vitamin E called gamma-tocopherol and a variety of plant chemicals such as flavanols that, at least in a test tube have potent antioxidant properties.

What wasn't terribly clear was how 'bioavailable' these were. Bioavailability is how much of a particular nutrient, or group of nutrients, is capable of being absorbed and used by our bodies. And it's important because no matter how many beneficial nutrients a food contains, if our bodies can't absorb and use them they are not much use.

In an attempt to discover the bioavailability of the antioxidant compounds in pecans the researchers devised a clever study to measure this in sixteen healthy men and women at various points in the twenty-four hours after eating a meal containing pecans, or a meal the same in every other respect but without pecans. What they found was that antioxidant capacity rose significantly in those who consumed the pecan meal. Meanwhile the oxidation of LDL cholesterol – remember that's the human equivalent of rusting and a key contributor to the development of heart disease – decreased by a third.

These are all encouraging pointers to the potential value of putting pecans on the menu. But in recent years there's been widespread recognition that there's more to cardiovascular disease (CVD) than dodgy blood fat levels. It's now recognised that CVD lies at the far end of a spectrum of conditions that doctors call cardiometabolic disease that begins earlier in life with insulin resistance (when the body can't use the hormone insulin properly), and then progresses to metabolic syndrome or pre-diabetes, type 2 diabetes, heart disease and stroke.

So what might be the effects of pecans on those tell-tale early cardiometabolic 'markers', such as blood glucose, insulin levels, blood pressure, inflammation, and the elasticity of the arteries? To find out, researchers from Tufts University in Boston in the US looked at what happened when twenty-six men and women, at high risk of developing cardiometabolic disease by dint of being aged 45+ and overweight or obese with that stubborn potentially harmful fat around the middle, added pecans to their diet in a randomised, controlled trial.

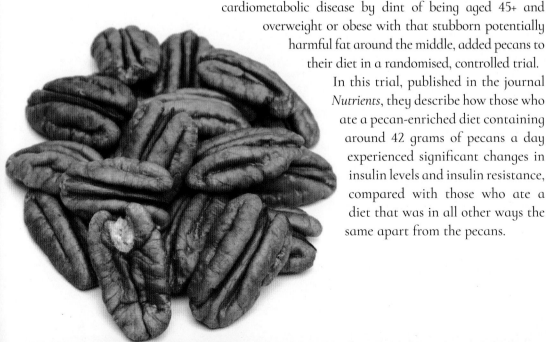

In this trial, published in the journal *Nutrients*, they describe how those who ate a pecan-enriched diet containing around 42 grams of pecans a day experienced significant changes in insulin levels and insulin resistance, compared with those who ate a diet that was in all other ways the same apart from the pecans.

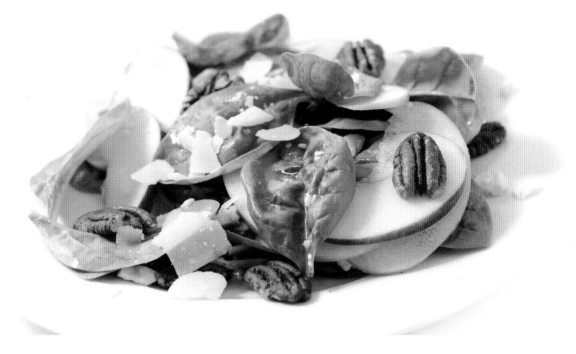

The participants on the pecan-enriched diet also experienced a significant improvement in the function of the insulin producing cells in the pancreas and in other markers of a high risk of cardiometabolic disease. An intriguing result, especially as it was obtained after just four weeks of putting pecans on the menu.

BRAIN AND NERVOUS SYSTEM

If there is little research on pecans' specific benefits for the heart, there is even less on their effects on the brain and nervous system. Still, we know that what is good for the heart is good for the brain, and those proanthocyanidin plant chemicals that pecans are so rich in have been found to help thwart age-related cognitive decline. So could pecans help protect against memory loss in later life? We simply don't know the answer to this as, so far, scientists haven't investigated the effects of pecan consumption on the ageing brain either in animals or humans. However, given that research shows that a diet rich in nuts, fruit and vegetables may help maintain cognitive health, sprinkling a handful of pecan nuts over your morning porridge is not going to do your brain any harm and could possibly do it some good.

DID YOU KNOW?

Pecan kernels aren't the only part of these nuts to have health benefits. Extracts of pecan shells reduce alcohol-induced liver damage – at least in rats. Other research suggests that pecan shell extracts can combat cell damage caused by cyclophosphamide, a chemotherapy drug used to treat leukaemia and other forms of cancer.

IN THE KITCHEN

Add to other nuts of your choice for snacking on raw.

Include in home-made muesli and granola mixes or add to smoothies.

Sprinkle over salads – they are great as an alternative to walnuts in French Roquefort salad with the cheese of the same name, or try them with shaved parmesan, spinach and apple – delicious.

Pour over melted butter or oil and spices (e.g. cayenne, cinnamon, cumin) or savoury sauces of your choice (e.g. Tabasco and/or Worcestershire).

Toast, roast or dry fry and serve as a snack at barbecues, drinks parties and other nibbling occasions.

For a sweet version mix together sugar, salt, cinnamon, cloves and nutmeg.

Add to cakes, biscuits and breads.

IT'S YOUR CHOICE...

To maximise nutrient benefits experts recommend storing in a cool place and consuming pecans unprocessed to maximise their nutrient benefits. Why? They are especially high in rancidity prone PUFAs.

PINE NUTS

Pinus Spp.

A part from the ubiquitous pesto sauce we usually consume pine nuts in relatively small quantities meaning that they have, to a large extent, escaped inclusion in the large, well-regarded studies on nuts and health that feature elsewhere. But these days they are causing quite a stir on account of their unique and unusual nutrient content which, experts suggest, could help ease inflammation, control weight, improve blood fat profile, increase the body's ability to handle insulin and more.

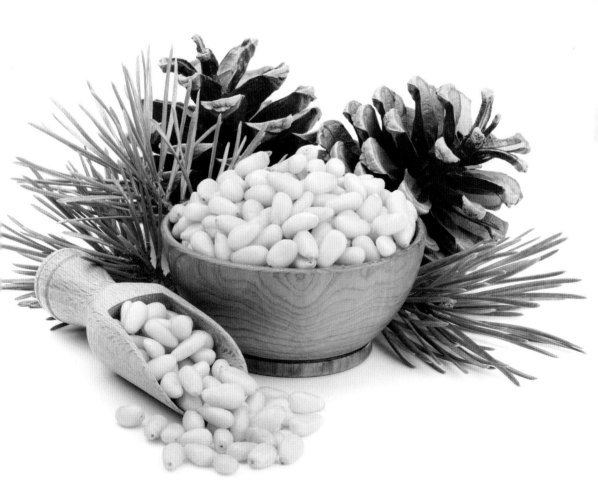

It seems that we humans have enjoyed a handful of these edible seeds since Palaeolithic times. Fast forward some millennia and Spanish explorers in the sixteenth century found Native American Indians eating them raw and roasted as well as using them ground in a type of meal.

The most common pine nuts in Europe are the small, cream-coloured, elongated oval seeds of the Mediterranean or Italian Stone Pine, a tall pine tree with an umbrella-shaped canopy of leaves recognisable to anyone who has travelled in Provence, Italy and the Middle East. These are, however, just one among twenty-nine other varieties – including Korean pine nuts which are currently attracting research attention – consumed as foods all with a similar although not identical nutrient profile.

A RARE PROFILE

With between 10 and 34 per cent of protein plus dietary fibre, B vitamins, different forms of vitamin E, the minerals calcium, copper, iron, potassium, magnesium, phosphorus, manganese and zinc, the plant sterol, camposterol, and a variety of phytonutrients, including the antioxidant gallic and ellagic acids, pine nuts are certainly not short on nutrients.

One of their most standout features is their rich and unusual fatty acid content. As well as the more familiar MUFAs and PUFAs, oleic acid and linoleic acid, respectively for science nerds out there, pine nuts contain a variety of unique and rare PUFAs. One of these in particular called pinolenic acid, which accounts for 14–19 per cent of their fat content, is attracting much interest from researchers on account of its potential health effects.

INFLAMMATION AND IMMUNITY

One of the most extensive studies of pinolenic acid is a research review carried out by scientists from the UK's Southampton University published in the *Journal of Functional Foods*. The researchers drew together the findings of several studies looking at the effects of pinolenic acid from Korean and Siberian pine nut oils, which are especially rich in this particular compound.

One of their most interesting findings in light of the fact that inflammation is now regarded as such a key player in chronic disease, is that pinolenic acid appears to lower the production of inflammatory chemicals, at least in cells in a test tube and in lab animals.

Another important finding, also in animals, is the ability of pine nut oil to boost levels of immune system chemicals, although the researchers point out this didn't hold true in all studies. Of course, the human body is a complicated organism and, as you are well aware by now, test tube and animal studies don't always carry over into benefits for us humans. But these findings do suggest the researchers' interest in pine nuts is not misplaced.

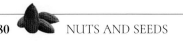

WEIGHT AND APPETITE CONTROL

Pine nut oil is much hyped for its supposed hunger suppressing qualities, although it has to be said that most research is still at too early a stage to draw any very meaningful conclusions. More specifically, in the test tube, Korean pine nut oil seems to boost levels of a key gut hormone involved in digesting protein and fat, known to play an important role in triggering feelings of satiety (aka feeling full) and switching off appetite. So how does this play out outside the lab?

One of the few studies to consider this question, was a small randomised, double-blind crossover trial, of eighteen overweight post-menopausal women from the Netherlands, and reported in *Lipids in Health and Disease*. Those who took a capsule of a proprietary product, PinnoThin, containing 3 grams of PUFAs derived from Korean pine-nut oil with a light breakfast had higher levels of this hormone, known as CCK short for cholecystokinin, compared with women who took an olive oil placebo. They also had higher levels of another hormone GLP-1, involved in regulating blood glucose levels. The women experienced a 29 per cent downturn in the desire to eat as well as a 36 per cent fall in the food they ate at the next meal.

Before you get too excited about this and start scoffing any old pine nuts morning, noon and night, it's worth noting that this was one small commercial study looking at a particular product containing Korean pine oil specifically. It's a finding that underlines the importance of provenance – and perhaps synergy with other nutrients – when it comes to drawing conclusions about the effects of food on health.

More recent research offers a clue as to the origin of these potential benefits. A Korean study published in *Nutrition Research and Practice* found that Korean pine nut oil may prevent the body from absorbing excess fat as well as boosting the ability of the liver to metabolise fats. Once again, it's just one small study and in mice at that,

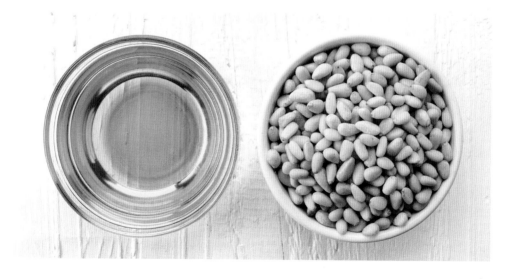

but it does provide a possible explanation as to how Korean pine nut oil and perhaps pinolenic acid may exert a positive effect.

BLOOD FATS AND INSULIN

What about other aspects of so-called metabolic health – that is, levels of blood fats, insulin, blood glucose and so on? Well, according to the Southampton scientists, Korean pine-nut oil and its extracts have the ability to lower 'bad' LDL cholesterol. Other studies, meanwhile, suggest that they may also lower levels of blood glucose and enhance the body's ability to use insulin effectively – in other words they help combat insulin resistance, which is a forerunner of type 2 diabetes. Again these are test tube and animal studies so it's not possible to draw definitive conclusions on how it affects humans, but it's certainly worth keeping an eye out for future studies.

CANCER

When it comes to cancer the story with regard to fatty acids is a complicated one. Some PUFAs seem to have the ability to block cancer development, while others appear to fuel it. So what role might pinolenic acid have to play? In a Taiwanese study published in the journal *Food Chemistry*, adding pinolenic acid to breast-cancer cells in

PINE NUT SYNDROME – A BITTER TASTE IN THE MOUTH

In recent years, doctors have reported a strange phenomenon called Pine Mouth – aka pine-nut related dysgeusia or Pine Nut Syndrome. This is a temporary taste disturbance, which results in what sufferers describe as a constant intensely bitter and/or metallic taste in the mouth one to three days after consuming pine nuts. Other reported symptoms include dry mouth, a sensation of swollen tonsils, nausea, headache, diarrhoea and vomiting. Fortunately, symptoms generally subside within a week or two and there appear to be no long term ill effects. The culprits are pine nuts from the species of *Pinus armandii*, Chinese White Pine, rather than the more familiar *Pinus pinea*.

As yet what causes Pine Mouth is unknown but it is thought to be linked to an inherited variation in bitter taste perception. Scientists writing in the journal *Chemical Biodiversity* recently tried to identify the potential offending ingredients by analysing the nutrient profile especially the content and the composition of fatty acids, vitamin E compounds, and amino acids in twenty-two different species of pine nuts. However, they were unable to reach a clear conclusion as to the culprit.

a test tube reduced their ability to move about and to invade other tissues, although it didn't stop them from proliferating, suggesting that pinolenic acid could possibly help to slow cancer spread. This led the researchers to conclude that it has possibilities as an anti-cancer agent. However, as with all such studies, it's important to exercise extreme caution and bear in mind that this was a test tube study. Nevertheless, it does add weight to a potentially promising picture.

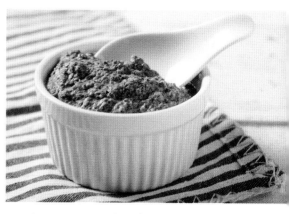

What might all this mean for us? Well, it certainly provides a cautious thumbs up for pine nuts and their oil, meaning that you could do worse than pop a packet of pine nuts or a bottle of pine nut oil in your kitchen cupboard or fridge.

IN THE KITCHEN

Add fresh raw pine nuts to salads, smoothies, muesli, granolas and other cereal based dishes.

Whizz up a handful of fresh pine nuts with basil, olive oil and a hard grated cheese, such as Parmesan or Pecorino, for a classic pesto and to top pasta or courgetti, fish, new potatoes, roasted vegetables tray bakes and savoury snacks deilate such as cheese straws and biscuits.

A dollop of pesto also goes down a treat swirled into a bowl of soup or on top of pizza. For a change why not substitute spinach for basil leaves?

Toast or stir fry pine nuts and sprinkle over salads, soups, yogurts, courgetti (courgette spaghetti) or vegetable-stuffed pancakes.

Chop and add to stuffing for poultry or vegetables such as Portobello mushrooms

Sugar glaze or drizzle honey over pine nuts and use in dessert recipes such as sweet fruit tarts or baked peaches.

Drizzle – preferable cold pressed – pine nut oil over salads, bakes and other dishes.

IT'S YOUR CHOICE...

Want to maximise the antioxidant capacity of those health promoting polyphenols in pine nuts? Stir fry briefly at a low temperature 50°C (122°F). Stir frying for longer (20 minutes) and at a high temperature 150°C (302°F) causes levels of polyphenols to plummet.

PISTACHIOS

Pistacia vera

Thanks to an exceptional nutrient profile the aptly named pistachios – the word from the ancient Greek pistakion simply means 'green nuts' – are big players in the tree nut world increasingly hailed for their potential to help control weight and fend off type 2 diabetes and possibly reduce the risk of heart disease.

Humans have eaten pistachios for more than 6,000 years with traces found at archaeological sites in Afghanistan and south eastern Iran. They were widely cultivated in the ancient Persian Empire. And, according to legend, the Queen of Sheba had a crop of pistachios earmarked for her own personal use. Meanwhile the Assyrians and ancient Greeks used them in medicines, as aphrodisiacs and as dyes.

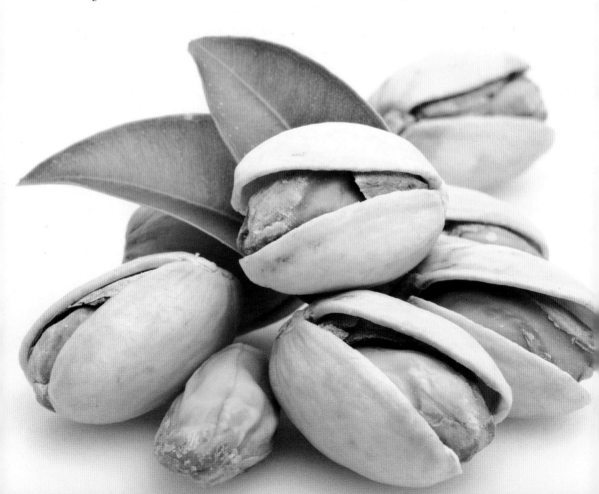

Lower in calories and fat than most other nuts, pistachios are packed with protein, the MUFA, oleic acid also found in olive oil, as well as PUFAs linked with a healthier heart and arteries. They are also richer in fibre than other nuts as well as having the highest levels of cholesterol-lowering plant sterols. With a wealth of minerals including calcium, magnesium, phosphorus and potassium and vitamins A, E, C, K and some B vitamins that all adds up to a potentially powerful nutritional punch.

But that's not all. Pistachios also contain a host of antioxidant, anti-inflammatory phytonutrients. These include resveratrol, also found in grape skins, peanuts and red wine, catechins, found in green tea, and lutein and zeaxanthin, yellow pigmented plant compounds found in kale, spinach and other green leafy veg that have been linked to better eye health. All these attributes have earned them a well-deserved place in the nutritional league table as one of the top fifty antioxidant foods, so let's look more closely at those potential health benefits.

HEART

The credentials of pistachios for a healthy heart are well established in studies looking at nuts in general. But do they have any benefits specifically? An overview of studies published in the journal *Acta Biomedica* found that pistachios were linked with reduced levels both total and 'bad' LDL cholesterol as well as increasing levels of 'good' HDL' cholesterol. They also were linked with lower levels of other blood fats, triglycerides, and had benefits overall for the blood fat profile including that crucial ratio of 'bad' LDL to 'good' HDL cholesterol. Just as importantly, the researchers could find no evidence of any unfavourable changes in levels of blood fats.

BEYOND GOOD AND BAD CHOLESTEROL

In recent years scientists have begun to refine their thinking around cholesterol and are now looking beyond the total, 'bad' LDL and 'good' HDL measurements. One of their most important discoveries is that certain LDL cholesterol particles, known as small dense lipoprotein particles are linked to an increased risk of type 2 diabetes and heart disease, so you don't want too many of those in your bloodstream.

So a clinical trial published in the journal *Nutrition, Metabolism and Cardiovascular Diseases* of fifty-four men and women with pre-diabetes, which showed that adding 57 grams of pistachio nuts, half roasted and half roasted and salted, significantly lowered levels of those small, dense lipoprotein particles shifting their blood fats in a direction less likely to cause furred, narrowed arteries is an intriguing finding.

In fact, say the researchers, their study showing that regular consumption of pistachio nuts has beneficial effects on these newly emerging risk factors for heart disease, even though it has little or no effect on the classic risk 'markers', could help explain why eating nuts is linked with a lower risk both of developing heart disease and of dying from it. The study was funded by the American Pistachio Growers (USA) and a group of pistachio farms, so a pinch of salt is perhaps needed. However, it does fit in with the growing body of research suggesting that nuts can improve heart health.

BLOOD PRESSURE

In another trial, one of relatively few to look specifically at the effects of nuts on blood pressure, researchers measured the effects of pistachios both on this as well as the elasticity of the arteries in ten men and eighteen women, all of whom were otherwise healthy except for raised levels of 'bad' LDL cholesterol. After two weeks eating a typical Western diet, they spent four weeks on the low-fat diet at one time recommended by the American Heart Association for heart health. This was followed by another four weeks in which they snacked on one serving a day of pistachios and a further four weeks in which they ate two servings of pistachios (supplying 10 per cent and 20 per cent of calories from pistachios respectively) in place of baked potato crisps and pretzels. All the meals were carefully calorie controlled.

At the end of each four-week period, participants had their blood pressure and other heart health 'markers' measured. Unlike when you have your BP measured at the surgery, the researchers didn't just measure BP at rest, they also measured it when the participants were under stress. And what better way to pile on the stress than to make people do a maths test or immerse a hand in icy water?

Both the pistachio-supplemented diets significantly reduced systolic blood pressure – the top figure, remember, that reflects the highest blood pressure when the heart is contracting, which gives the best clue to the risk of having a stroke or heart attack. Interestingly this effect was greater in those who consumed one serving a day than those who consumed two servings a day of pistachios.

Meanwhile with two servings a day the researchers noted an improvement in the elasticity of the blood vessels and other measures of arterial health. It's a result that mirrors the results of another study published in *Nutrients* showing that pistachio nuts improved arterial stiffness and the ability of the inner lining of the arteries to respond to the demands of everyday life. Given the value of eating foods that potentially target lots of different risk factors for heart disease these findings suggest that pistachios deserve their increasing reputation for heart friendliness.

PRE-DIABETES AND DIABETES

Before type 2 diabetes kicks in there is a stage called pre-diabetes or 'metabolic syndrome'. This consists of a cluster of symptoms – high blood glucose, high levels of blood fats and high blood pressure – together with being overweight accompanied by

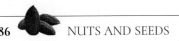

a large waist circumference – that classic apple shape, and insulin resistance, when the body produces but can't respond properly to the hormone insulin.

Reversing these and other 'markers' of pre-diabetes has become something of a holy grail for researchers as a way to halt or slow progress to type 2 diabetes. So the findings of the study already outlined above in respect of blood fat profile in people with pre-diabetes showing that putting pistachios on the menu significantly lowered blood glucose levels, insulin levels and other markers of insulin resistance is welcome.

But what if you already have diabetes? It seems that adding a couple of handfuls of pistachios a day to your diet could be a smart move, says an Iranian study. The researchers divided forty-eight people with type 2 diabetes into two groups. For the first twelve weeks one group was given two snacks each containing 25 grams of pistachios and asked to eat them every day. The second group received no nuts. At the end of this period both groups were tested on a variety of 'markers' for diabetes. Then after an eight-week gap the groups swapped over and the people in the second group were given the pistachio snacks.

The researchers found a marked downturn in levels of HbA1c, a marker of longer-term blood glucose control, as well as in fasting blood glucose (FBG) level in those who supplemented pistachios. Echoing the previously mentioned study, pistachio consumption also reduced systolic blood pressure, as well as lowering BMI – aka body mass index – and C-reactive protein (CRP), a measure of inflammation, although there was no effect on insulin resistance.

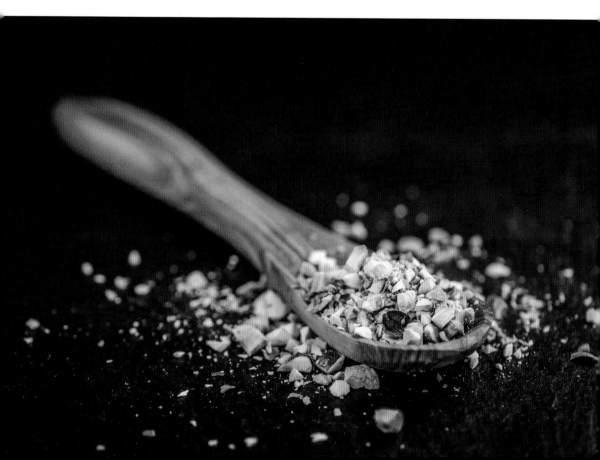

These two studies are included in an overview published in the journal *Critical Reviews in Food Science and Nutrition* looking at ways in which pistachios might benefit people with pre-diabetes and diabetes. The researchers conclude that putting 50-57 grams of pistachios a day on the menu (amounting to around 20 per cent of daily calorie intake) could positively influence glucose control in just one to four months. The reasons? In a word: synergy. They surmise the combined effects of MUFAs and PUFAs – plus the activity of specific phytochemicals in pistachios affect the action of molecules responsible for turning genes on and off as well as improving insulin sensitivity through a chemical 'pathway' linked with the development of diabetes.

PREGNANCY MATTERS

Before we leave diabetes, a word about the effects of pistachios on gestational diabetes (GD), a type of diabetes that strikes in pregnancy. Once considered merely a temporary blip that went away after pregnancy, in recent years researchers have taken it more seriously because women who develop it are now known to have a greater risk of developing type 2 diabetes in later life. This makes the results of a Spanish study published in the journal *PLoS One* showing that a Mediterranean diet with added pistachio nuts helped to reduce the risk of GD welcome.

The study included 874 women with normal blood glucose levels at the start, who were allocated to eat either a Mediterranean diet supplemented with extra virgin olive oil (EVOO) and pistachios, or a standard diet with a limited fat intake. As well as reducing the risk of developing GD, the study found that adding pistachio nuts to the diet significantly reduced the need to treat GD with insulin as well as lowering the risk of prematurity, emergency caesarean section, injury to the tissues during birth and increasing the likelihood of having a normal weight baby. Interesting findings, which if you're pregnant or planning a pregnancy, could be worth factoring in when you make food choices.

WEIGHT

Worried about putting on weight? Rather than piling on the kilos or increasing the risk of becoming overweight, pistachios may aid weight control. How? Their relatively low calorie count plus their fibre, protein and fat content, together with their crunchy texture is thought to help satiety – that feeling of fullness that stops you eating when you've had enough and reduces the urge to snack.

And here's a tip. If you opt for pistachios as your go-to snack, choose them shell-on. Studies show that eating pistachios in their shells can help keep down the calorie count. In fact simply looking at those empty shells seems to help curb appetite. In a study published in the aptly named journal *Appetite*, workers who left the shells on their desk consumed 18 per cent fewer calories than those who threw the shells away.

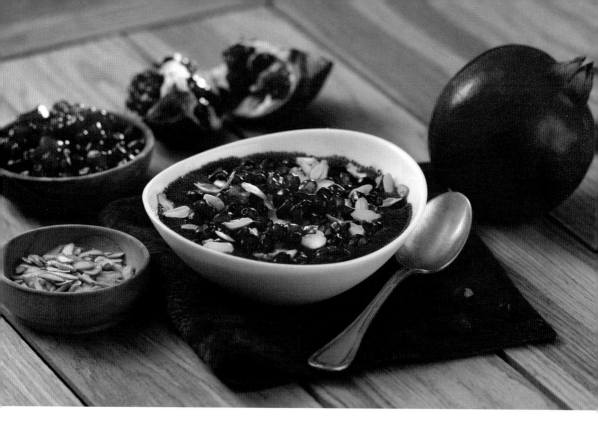

GUT BACTERIA

One way in which pistachios may exert beneficial effects on blood glucose and type 2 diabetes is by their influence on gut bacteria. While both pistachios and almonds seem to have benefits, it seems pistachios may have a slight edge when it comes to helping create a healthy microbiome. In a 2014 US study published in the *British Journal of Nutrition*, researchers found that pistachio consumption increased the number of butyrate-producing bacteria in the gut in sixteen volunteers. Butyrate is a short-chain fatty acid (SCFA) that has been linked with better gut health.

In another study published in *The Journal of Nutritional Biochemistry* researchers found that in thirty-nine people with pre-diabetes, eating pistachio nuts resulted in significant beneficial changes in secondary metabolites (chemicals produced by the action of gut bacteria) measured in the urine, all of which are linked with the disturbances in body chemistry associated with insulin resistance and Type 2 diabetes.

DID YOU KNOW?

In a 2018 study published in the journal *Molecules*, for example, researchers found that an extract derived from pistachio shells helped stop the development of blood vessels that serve cancer cells as well as encouraging cancer cells to commit suicide (apoptosis) in breast cancer cells in the test tube suggesting this is an area ripe for more research.

Incidentally, if you happen to visit Sicily on holiday, stock up on pistachio nuts. Researchers have found that the Sicilian variety of Pistachio Valle del Platani, much prized by chefs and foodies, is rich in the omega-7 fatty acid palmitoleic acid, which is attracting interest for its potential beneficial effects on insulin resistance and other aspects of health.

IN THE KITCHEN

The good news is that pistachios retain their nutritional benefits even after cooking. Here's how to add some pistachio-power to your diet:

Snack on pistachios instead of crisps and other less nutritious snacks.

Add chopped shelled pistachios to stir fries, soups, salads, yoghurts and dips such as houmous.

Mix with other nuts and seeds for an extra nutrient boost – for example chopped pistachios and pomegranate seeds make a great topping for a lentil soup.

Boost nutrient value and reduce GI by adding chopped or ground pistachios to pasta, mashed potatoes and rice.

Chop and add to salsas, marinades and rubs.

Top puddings such as chia pudding with chopped pistachios and fruit.

IT'S YOUR CHOICE...

To lower the blood glucose boosting effects of foods such as rice and pasta add a handful of chopped pistachios. The reason? Pistachios have a low glycaemic index or GI, a measure of the effect of different foods on the surge of blood glucose that happens when we eat. Pasta and rice on the other hand have a high GI. Research shows that adding pistachios helps to counteract this. Pasta and pesto: a match made in heaven.

PUMPKIN SEEDS

Cucurbita pepo/maxima

With a complex mixture of proteins, fatty acids, antioxidant vitamins, minerals and plant chemicals pumpkin seeds are fast gaining a reputation for helping bladder problems, diabetes and more. Some of their more notable nutrients include gamma-tocopherol, a type of vitamin E thought to be especially effective in combatting inflammation as well as phytoestrogens, plant chemicals with a weak oestrogen-like effect.

First domesticated some 10,000 years ago, pumpkins and their seeds were staple foods in the Americas long before European colonisation. Today they remain a popular snack in Greece and other Mediterranean countries, raw, roasted and/or salted or as an ingredient in bread, cereals, salads and cakes.

With such a favourable nutrient profile it's not surprising that pumpkin seeds and their oil are currently attracting a great deal of research interest for their potential health benefits. These include helping improve bladder and prostate problems, reducing the risk of cardiometabolic problems – high levels of blood fats, high insulin and blood glucose – that increase the risk of type two diabetes, heart disease, stroke, cancer and more. So how does the science add up?

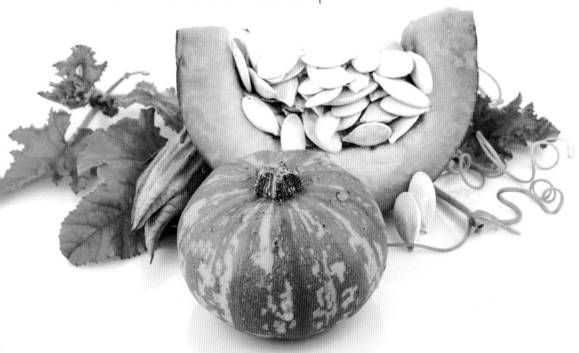

BLADDER

Pumpkin seeds have a reputation in traditional medicine from Central Europe to the Caribbean for helping ease bladder problems, especially those caused by BPH – aka benign prostatic hyperplasia – that is enlargement of the prostate. The bane of life for many men aged 50+, BPH causes a catalogue of symptoms including frequency, as the term suggests a frequent or urgent need to urinate, difficulty urinating, dribbling, a weak urine stream and sleep disturbance caused by having to get up and down constantly at night to go to the loo. Unsurprisingly men with BPH often report a diminished quality of life.

Could pumpkin seeds ease symptoms help improve matters? Well it seems that they may help to tone the bladder as well as helping to block an enzyme involved in hormone metabolism which helps build and strengthen the bladder muscles and relaxing the urinary sphincter so decreasing frequency of urination. In line with this, studies both in the lab and in humans suggest they could be of benefit for bladder problems caused either by BPH or other reasons, although it's hard to draw firm conclusions because of variations in quality, size and duration of studies.

At the time of writing, there are only three randomised, controlled trials, considered the gold standard when making judgements about treatments. What do these tell us? According to an Italian review looking at the state of the science as it stood in 2016, pumpkin seeds can improve symptoms of BPH and quality of life. So, although the researchers concede that more good quality clinical trials are needed, at least some of the money appears to be on pumpkin seeds – or their derivatives – for treating BPH.

OVERACTIVE BLADDER

It's not just bladder problems caused by BPH that pumpkin seeds seem to help. In a Japanese study published in the *Journal of Traditional and Complementary Medicine*, forty-five men and women, aged 41 to 80 years complaining of symptoms of an overactive bladder, took an extract of pumpkin seed oil. After twelve weeks the participants reported a significant improvement in symptoms such as day and night time frequency, urgency, and loss of bladder control caused by not making it to the loo in time. Of course, a single study of forty-five people isn't a lot to go on so, as so often, it's a matter of more research being needed. However if you suffer with an overactive bladder it may not be a bad idea to keep a bottle of pumpkin seed oil in your cupboard to include in your salad dressing.

Another study, this time Slovakian, also published in the *Journal of Alternative and Complementary Medicine* looked at the effects of a proprietary pumpkin-seed and flax-seed extract on stress incontinence, leakage of urine caused by coughing, laughing, sneezing or any exertion such as jumping, running, dancing and even sometimes walking. The study, which included eighty-six women aged from 32 to 88 years with mild-to-moderate stress incontinence, found that this preparation resulted in a 30 per cent improvement in mild stress incontinence and 35 per cent in those with moderate stress incontinence after just twelve weeks.

The study also found that the number of times women needed to urinate improved by 40 per cent in those with mild symptoms and 26 per cent in those with moderate symptoms. Meanwhile night-time urinary frequency was improved by 64 per cent and 54 per cent in those with mild and moderate symptoms respectively. Just a single study again, but one that suggests further research could be worthwhile.

BLOOD GLUCOSE, CHOLESTEROL, WEIGHT AND MORE

Pumpkins themselves are gaining a fair old reputation as functional foods to treat and prevent diabetes thanks to their ability to lower blood glucose. But what about the seeds? Test-tube studies and studies in animals, suggest that pumpkin-seed extracts could indeed lower blood glucose. In one Indian study published in the *Journal of Traditional and Complementary Medicine*, for example, blood glucose dropped by 26 per cent in lab rats with mild diabetes and by almost 40 per cent in those with severe diabetes, results on a par with diabetes medication. The reasons? The combined effect of the cocktail of proteins, carbohydrates and plant chemicals in pumpkin seeds, suggest the researchers.

Other research also in rats, published in the *North American Journal of Medical Science*, reveals that pumpkin seeds mixed with either flaxseeds or purslane, a bitter wild herb that often crops up in wild greens or *horta* on taverna menus in Greece, lower cholesterol, protect the kidneys and boost immunity. Just as intriguingly, the rats who ate the purslane and pumpkin-seed mix lost weight, something the researchers suggest is attributable to the pumpkin seeds. It's a fascinating study and yet another example of the synergy between nutrients as well as a further plus point for eating the Mediterranean way. But of course we do need some studies in humans before coming to any firm conclusions.

Meanwhile another Indian study published in the journal *Archives of*

Physiology and Biochemistry in which scientists examined the potential effects of pumpkin-seed oil in rats, this time fed a high fat diet, on body weight and blood fat profile, found again that pumpkin-seed oil reduced weight and also changed chemical 'markers' of a poor blood fat profile and of inflammation. As you're well aware by now, however, a handful of small studies in rats are a far cry from studies in human beings, but they are a start – and a promising one at that – so it's worth keeping an eye out for further studies.

BREAST CANCER

You may have seen claims that pumpkin seeds can help protect against breast cancer. But to be honest it's far too early to argue this with any great certainty. There are good reasons to suggest that pumpkin seeds could have an effect as, as well as being rich in fibre, they contain fibre-linked plant oestrogens – or phytoestrogens – called lignans that mimic the effects of oestrogen.

A German case-control study (a type of observational study see page 125 for what this sort of study is) published in the journal *Nutrition and Cancer* which examined data on the diets of 2,884 women with breast cancer, and 5,509 women without the disease, found that both high and low consumption of pumpkin seeds (as well as soya beans and sunflower seeds) was linked with a significantly lower breast cancer risk compared to no consumption.

Studies like this come pretty low down on the pecking order of research so it's not possible to draw any great conclusion from this. However, it does support the finding of test-tube research, also published in the journal *Nutrition and Cancer*, showing that pumpkin-seed extract can influence receptors, structures on the surface cells that allow chemicals, including oestrogen that fuels some types of breast cancer, into cells a bit like a lock and key. The results, say the German researchers who made this finding, 'could highlight a potential role of pumpkin seed's lignans in breast cancer prevention and/or treatment.'

WOUND-HEALING

Finally, even if you don't eat the seeds, applying pumpkin-seed oil topically could have benefits. In a study, cold-pressed pumpkin-seed oil helped to encourage faster wound-healing, although again in rats.

So what's the verdict? The science is certainly tantalising and suggests that pumpkin seeds could have considerable promise. Whether this will be fulfilled remains to be seen so again, as with other nuts and seeds, we will have to wait and see. But if you like the flavour it could certainly be worth keeping some pumpkin seeds and pumpkin-seed oil on standby in your cupboard or fridge.

IN THE KITCHEN

PUMPKIN SEEDS

Snack on roasted whole or shelled seeds, either alone or with other seeds or nuts (sesame, sunflower and linseeds go especially well with pumpkin seeds) or dried fruit.

Add to muesli and granola.

Sprinkle over salads, soups, stews and/or stir fries.

Add to pasta sauces for a delicious nutty crunch.

Use instead of pine nuts for a tasty take on pesto sauce.

Use to top homemade bread and rolls or add to biscuit and cake mixes.

For variety roast your own pumpkin seeds adding seasonings such as chilli, cumin, paprika, tamari sauce, sumac, five spice mix, za'tar, or if you want a sweet taste, brown sugar or honey.

PUMPKIN-SEED OIL

Use gently warmed or cold but don't fry – it has a low smoke point 100°C (212°F).

Mix with vinegar and herbs (purslane if you can get it) for salad dressing.

Drizzle over stir fried vegetables, rice and pasta instead of sesame oil.

IT'S YOUR CHOICE...

Buying pumpkin seed oil? Go for a cold-pressed toasted variety. Research suggests that any loss of nutrients is minimal and it is less likely to go rancid.

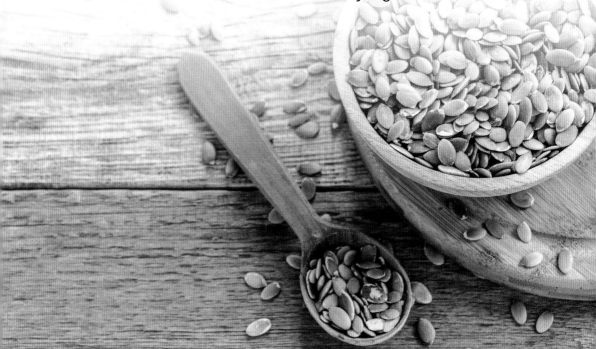

QUINOA

Chenopodium quinoa Willd

Rich in fibre, vitamins B, C and E and minerals as well as numerous antioxidant and anti-inflammatory phytochemicals, which as we've seen elsewhere have been linked to helping prevent a wide range of diseases, quinoa seeds are gaining a growing reputation for their potential health benefits.

Quinoa is a relative of spinach and beets. Native to the Andes, it is one of the world's oldest known foods cultivated for around 7,000 years. There are more than 3,000 varieties both cultivated and wild. But although all parts of the plant can be eaten, it is the seeds, known by the Incas as 'the golden grain', that in recent years have attracted a flurry of attention thanks to their exceptional nutrient profile.

Gluten-free, quinoa seeds are the only plant food to contain all twenty amino acids, the building blocks of protein. These include nine 'essential' amino acids, so called because our bodies can't produce them. This provides a protein value similar

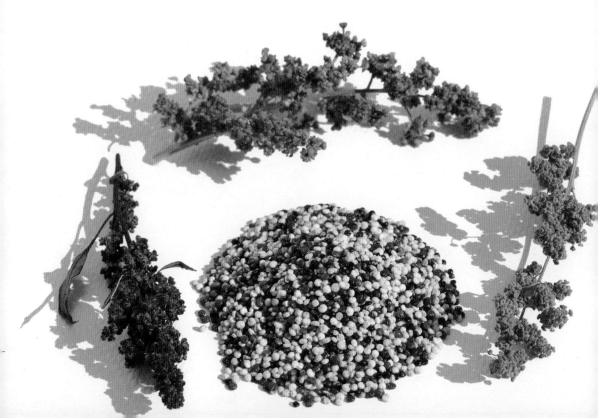

to casein, one of the main proteins in milk, something which makes them close to the ideal protein balance recommended by the UN Food and Agriculture Organisation (FAO) and a good choice for vegans.

Perhaps it's no surprise then that the FAO is promoting quinoa as part of a strategy to encourage cultivation of traditional and forgotten crops to bolster food security for current and future generations. Let's find out some more about quinoa's promise on the health front.

HEART

Several animal studies suggest that quinoa seeds can improve the blood fat profile – that is lower cholesterol and other harmful blood fats called triglycerides, which are also linked with a higher risk of heart disease. But what happens in people? It's early days to draw definitive conclusions but there are hints that point in the same direction.

For example, in a Brazilian study, scientists looked at the effects of consuming cereal bars containing quinoa for thirty days on twenty-two students aged from 18-45 years. At the end of the study they had a significant reduction in cholesterol levels. What's more, 56.7 per cent of them also had lower blood glucose levels, 42 per cent weighed less and 40 per cent had lower blood pressure. Meanwhile in one of the few randomised controlled trials published in *Current Developments in Nutrition*, Australian scientists asked a group of people aged 18 to 65 to add quinoa seeds to their normal diet. Those who needed it were coached in how to cook quinoa and issued with recipes. At the end of the study participants who consumed 50 grams of white, organic quinoa seeds had significantly lower levels of those harmful triglyceride blood fats compared with those who consumed 25 grams of quinoa seeds or a placebo.

All the participants in this trial – sixty-four in all – had a BMI of more than 25, meaning that they had a higher risk of problems such as heart disease, type 2 diabetes and stroke, so another finding that those who ate 50 grams of quinoa also had a 70 per cent lower prevalence of metabolic syndrome, which predisposes towards a greater risk of these conditions, is especially welcome. The message? If you're overweight and concerned about your blood fat profile you could do worse than put quinoa on the menu.

What accounts for these potential benefits? As outlined above, quinoa seeds contain a wealth of heart-friendly fats and are also packed with other nutrients such as fibre, potassium, magnesium and several different types of vitamin E that have been found to have benefits for the heart, plus an especially hefty dose of polyphenols, with twenty-three detected in them so far.

As with other nuts and seeds, it's almost certainly the synergy between these nutrients that accounts for quinoa's potential benefits. But two plant chemicals are worth flagging up. The first is quercetin, also found in onions, kale, leeks, broccoli, apples, tea, capers and blueberries, which has, according to a review in the journal

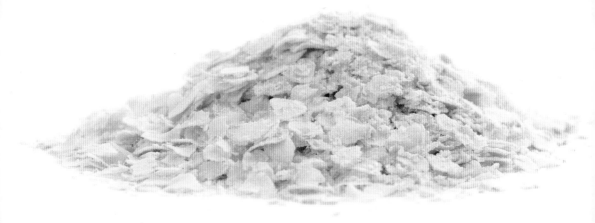

Mini reviews in medical chemistry, 'tremendous cardioprotective properties'. These include, according to a systematic review and meta-analysis published in the *Journal of the American Heart Association*, an ability to increase the elasticity of arteries and lower blood pressure.

The second is a natural fatty compound called squalene, which is involved in cholesterol synthesis and helps combat oxidative stress while increasing levels of 'good' HDL cholesterol, at least in mice. So says research published in the journal *PLoS One*. Interestingly, squalene is also found in olives and, as an ingredient of extra-virgin olive oil, is thought to be one of the melange of nutrients that could help contribute the health benefits of a Mediterranean diet.

WEIGHT AND DIABETES

If you've got this far, the fact that we are facing soaring levels of type 2 diabetes will not have escaped your notice. And, as you probably also recognise, this type of diabetes doesn't come on suddenly. It's preceded by years of high levels of blood glucose, plus increasing insulin resistance, when the body is unable to respond as it should to the hormone insulin – as well as high blood pressure and high levels of harmful blood fats, all driven by excess internal fat.

If we could find a way to somehow call a halt to this pre-diabetic state – aka metabolic syndrome – then it might also be possible to stop, or at least slow, its progression to type 2 diabetes. And according to the findings of a randomised controlled trial, published in the Spanish journal *Nutricion Hospitalaria*, quinoa could be a potentially valuable ally.

The researchers found that those who consumed quinoa, rather than a placebo, had a lower body-mass index or BMI, and felt fuller and more satisfied, something that is essential when you're trying to lose weight or more to the point fat. Admittedly this was a small study – just thirty people in all – but it does back up animal studies suggesting that quinoa can help lower high levels of blood glucose and help weight control.

In another Brazilian study, published in the *International Journal of Food Sciences and Nutrition*, when thrirty-five overweight, post-menopausal women consumed 25 grams of quinoa flakes daily instead of cornflakes, they had a lower BMI, lower total cholesterol, lower 'bad' LDL cholesterol, as well as lower levels of those harmful blood fats called triglycerides in the blood stream, at the end of four weeks.

There were no benefits on other markers of metabolic syndrome such as waist circumference, blood glucose levels and 'good' HDL cholesterol. But the women also had increased levels of a naturally produced antioxidant called glutathione, a shortage of which is linked with a whole host of health problems from cardiovascular disease to cancer and dementia. Again, it's a small study but with results like these it could be worth varying your breakfast cereal.

MENOPAUSE

Quinoa contains two phytoestrogens called isoflavones, which are thought to act like the female hormone, oestrogen, in the body. You might already have heard of these two compounds which go by the names daidzein and genistein, as they are also found in soya beans, albeit in smaller quantities. They have been linked with a lower risk of osteoporosis and with relief from hot flushes and night sweats, although the jury is still out on this one.

The colour of quinoa seeds is a clue to the content of these two nutrients. The highest daidzein level is found in red quinoa seeds from the high plains of Bolivia and Peru, while the highest genistein levels are found in black quinoa seeds. There aren't any specific studies on the value of quinoa seeds for these purposes but if you're coming up to, or have reached menopause already, it is perhaps something to bear in mind next time you're stocking up your store cupboard.

GUT

Some 6 per cent of the weight of quinoa grain consists of dietary fibre, great for healthy digestion, of course, and also for reducing cholesterol. But there's another benefit too and that is stimulating the development of healthy gut microbes. So could quinoa have particular benefits for gut health? A study reported in *Food and Function*, looking at the effects of quinoa on gut microbes, throws some interesting light on this. It found that quinoa seeds encouraged the production of short-chain fatty acids (SCFAs), which are thought to be needed for a healthy gut and other aspects of health. According to the researchers this suggests that quinoa may help rebalance gut bacteria and encourage gut health.

COELIAC DISEASE

One group who give quinoa a definite thumbs up are people with coeliac disease (CD). If you are one of them then of course cutting out gluten, found in wheat, rye and barley, is absolutely essential rather than a mere food fad. But going gluten-free can lead to nutrient deficiencies – people with CD are often short of fibre, B vitamins such as thiamine, riboflavin, niacin and folate as well as the minerals iron and calcium, for example. The reason for these deficiencies is partly because many people with CD don't consume enough grain products. Meanwhile many gluten-free products are low in essential nutrients like folate, iron and fibre.

In an attempt to remedy this, in a study reported in the *Journal of Human Nutrition and Dietetics,* specialist coeliac dietitians devised an alternative menu to the standard gluten-free diet, which did not meet recommended intakes fibre, thiamine, riboflavin, niacin folate, iron, or calcium. This included oats at breakfast time, a high-fibre brown-rice bread at lunch time and a side of quinoa in the evening, which they tested out on fifty people with CD. The change resulted in a much improved nutritional profile including significantly higher levels of protein, iron, calcium and fibre. Another study reported in the *American Journal of Gastroenterology* found that consuming 50 grams of quinoa a day for six weeks had a mild cholesterol-lowering effect in people with CD.

CANCER

Research published in the journal *Food Research International* meanwhile reveals that polysaccharides, carbohydrates found in quinoa, protect against liver cancer and breast cancer cells – at least in the test tube. Other research found that peptides, protein fragments, found in quinoa have anti-oxidant properties and can kill bowel cancer cells in a lab model of the gut. The researchers suggest: 'These proteins might be utilised as new ingredients in the development of functional foods or nutraceuticals

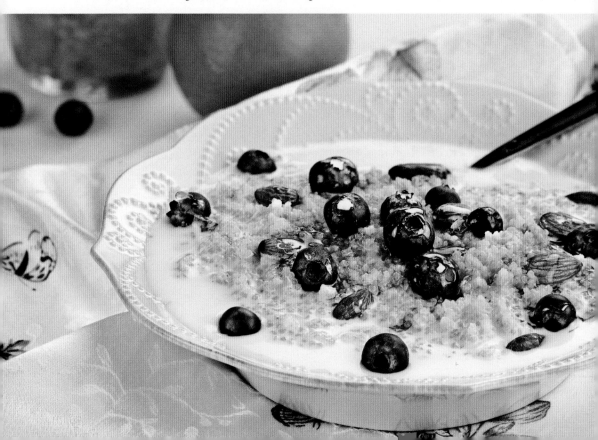

with the aim of reducing oxidative stress-associated diseases, including cancer.' Of course, as we all know, it's a long way from lab bench to the doctor's surgery. But it's certainly a pointer in the right direction.

> ## Take 3
>
> Three main varieties of quinoa are on sale. Try to vary your choices for maximum nutrients:
> 1. White quinoa – the best known and quickest cooking.
> 2. Red quinoa – great in salads as it doesn't disintegrate as easily as the other types.
> 3. Black quinoa – takes the longest time to cook and is much favoured by chefs for its distinctive sweet, earthy flavour and colour.

IN THE KITCHEN

Serve with a dash of olive oil and perhaps a few fresh herbs instead of rice to accompany curries, chili dishes, and stews.

Combine with dried fruit, cinnamon and milk in a breakfast bowl or make quinoa porridge for a nutritious start to the day.

Bulk out stir fries, stews and casseroles and burgers.

Add to salads or cold leftover roasted veg, such as butternut squash, add crumbled feta, cold or tinned fish, tofu or poultry for a speedy, nutritious lunch.

Use to stuff peppers, tomatoes, courgettes and other vegetables.

Stir into puddings.

Use in baking e.g. in breads or savoury or sweet muffins (you'll find lots of recipes online).

Note: Give quinoa a quick swoosh under running water before using to sluice away bitterness.

IT'S YOUR CHOICE...

Soak quinoa seeds for 12–14 hours, before fermenting with whey or allowing them to germinate for 30 hours and then cooking at 100°C (212°F) for 25 minutes. Why? To reduce levels of phytic acid, an 'anti-nutrient' found in cereals, legumes, oil seeds and nuts, which can block the absorption of minerals including iron, zinc calcium, magnesium and manganese and inhibit digestive enzymes.

SESAME SEEDS

Sesamun indicum

One of the most ancient cultivated plants, sesame is thought to be the first crop to have been grown for its edible oil. Some of the claimed benefits of sesame seeds include the ability to lower levels of harmful blood fats and blood pressure.

Sesame seeds are thought to have been used for near on 6,000 years, making them possibly the oldest known condiment. The magic words, 'Open sesame', famous from the Middle Eastern folk tales known in English as the Arabian Nights, and of course pantomimes, is said to refer to the way the seed pod explodes when ripe, scattering the seeds.

But is there magic for health in the nutrients found in sesame seeds? Antioxidant and anti-inflammatory, they are rich in protein, carbohydrates, fibre, B and E vitamins and minerals including calcium, iron and the trace element, selenium. They also contain phytochemicals, including the aptly named sesamin and

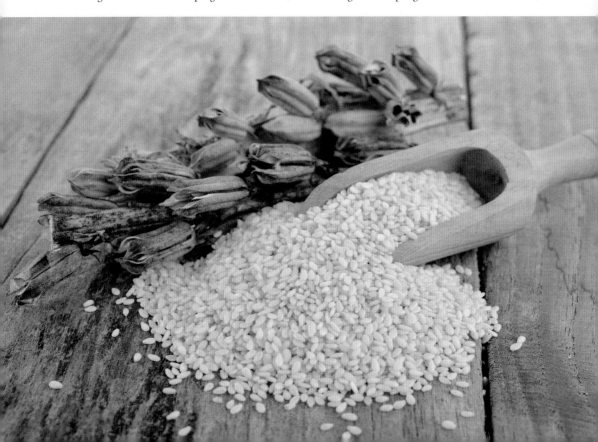

sesamol, and plant sterols, as well as an abundant supply of different fatty acids that are remarkably resistant to going rancid. All of which suggest sesame seeds and their oil could have distinct benefits for health. Let's examine some of them.

HEART

A host of lab and animal studies suggest that sesame seeds and their oil, together with the MUFAs, PUFAs, vitamin E, fibre, and phytochemicals they contain, could benefit the heart and arteries. A 2017 review published in the journal *Cureus* concluded that sesame oil can lower levels of 'bad' LDL cholesterol, while maintaining 'good' HDL cholesterol levels.

Meanwhile, an Iranian study published in the *Iranian Journal of Pharmacological Research* found that in diabetic lab rats (yes, there are such things) just seven weeks on a diet with added sesame seeds boosted the elasticity of their arteries. Stiff, inelastic arteries caused by high levels of blood glucose are a major culprit in the cardiovascular complications of diabetes. This was the first study to investigate the effects of sesame on the elasticity of the arteries in live animals rather than in a test tube, and the scientists surmise that their findings could aid the development of new, natural sesame-based treatments to prevent heart disease.

But what about the benefits of sesame seeds or oil for people? Truth to tell there aren't *that* many studies and certainly none is overwhelmingly convincing. But a 2018 systematic review (published in the journal *Critical Reviews in Food Science and Nutrition* concluded that sesame seeds and their derivatives could improve blood fat profile and blood pressure in people with high blood pressure and/or an unhealthy blood fat profile.

This review included seven clinical trials and, while the authors couldn't put their finger on the exact compounds responsible for these apparent benefits concluding that more higher quality clinical trials are needed to improve the evidence base, their findings are intriguing.

DIABETES AND PRE-DIABETES

In the past few years researchers have been getting pretty excited over the chief phytochemical in sesame seeds, sesamin, due to the fact that it appears to to restore the body's sensitivity to insulin. This is certainly the case in mice, according to a Chinese study published in the *Journal of the Science of Food and Agriculture*. Insensitivity to insulin – aka insulin resistance – is the main driver behind both type 2 diabetes and its precursor, pre-diabetes. So, could adding sesame seeds to your diet help prevent or treat diabetes? Unfortunately it's not possible to go that far. However, there is some research that suggests they could help with some of the consequences of diabetes.

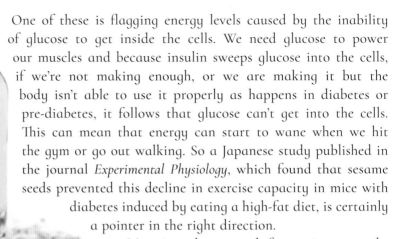

One of these is flagging energy levels caused by the inability of glucose to get inside the cells. We need glucose to power our muscles and because insulin sweeps glucose into the cells, if we're not making enough, or we are making it but the body isn't able to use it properly as happens in diabetes or pre-diabetes, it follows that glucose can't get into the cells. This can mean that energy can start to wane when we hit the gym or go out walking. So a Japanese study published in the journal *Experimental Physiology*, which found that sesame seeds prevented this decline in exercise capacity in mice with diabetes induced by eating a high-fat diet, is certainly a pointer in the right direction.

It's quite a long stretch from mice to people, so it's impossible to say if sesame seeds could have the same effect on human beings. But if you're looking for a pre-exercise snack you could perhaps do worse than having a crispbread with houmous made with a generous amount of tahini paste.

CANCER

But the benefits of sesamin apparently don't stop there. According to some studies, it could also have anti-cancer effects. Research from the Anderson Cancer Center in Houston, Texas, published in the journal *Molecular Cancer Research*, for example, found that sesamin works – much like a chemotherapy drug – to prevent the multiplication of several different kinds of cancer cells including those involved in leukaemia, multiple myeloma, another kind of blood cancer, colon, prostate, breast, pancreas, and lung cancer.

Meanwhile, a comprehensive review published the *European Journal of Pharmacology* points to the ability of sesamin to quell inflammation, cut off the blood supply to cancer cells, induce cells to commit suicide (apoptosis), suppress tumour development and prevent cancer cells from spreading, as being responsible for its potent anti-cancer effects. Great qualities you must admit, although clearly they need to be verified by further studies in animals and humans.

The very same properties that make sesamin such a potentially powerful weapon against cancer could, say the researchers, benefit other diseases. For example, its ability to suppress inflammation could make it useful in osteoarthritis and other inflammatory diseases.

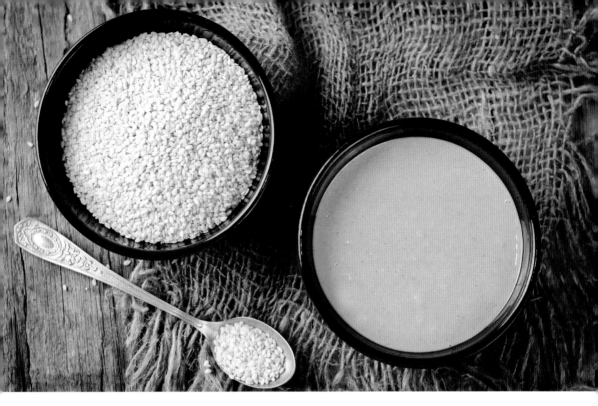

IN THE KITCHEN

SESAME SEEDS

Sprinkle raw or toasted seeds over salads, casseroles, stir-fries and noodle and rice dishes.

Garnish home-made loaves, rolls, bagels or muffins.

Add to muesli, granola or other breakfast cereal.

Use in risottos and pilaus.

Coat salmon and other firm fish with sesame seeds before frying or baking.

Add to energy bars, balls, smoothies.

Toast by placing in a dry frying pan and cooking, stirring occasionally until the seeds turn golden (3 to 5 mins). Alternatively spread on a baking tray and toast in the oven at 175°C (350°F) 8 to 15 mins.

TAHINI PASTE

Add tahini paste – made from ground sesame seeds – to humous. It also makes a great addition to salad dressings.

Take a leaf from famed chef Yotam Ottolenghi's book and keep some tahini sauce – a mix of tahini paste, water, crushed garlic, lemon juice and salt – in the fridge ready to drizzle over all manner of dishes from fish, to chicken to vegetable tray bakes.

He suggests thinning this with a dash of soy sauce, honey or cider vinegar, to give 'body to any bowl of greens'.

For a sweet treat add a swirl of tahini past to vanilla ice-cream, or to sweet makes and bakes such as chocolate brownies he says.

Use whole tahini (made by keeping some or all of the hull, and in some cases not toasting the seeds) spread on buttered toast or fresh bread.

Alternatively drizzle with honey, date or grape syrup, a practice traditional in Iraq and Turkey.

SESAME OIL

Use alone or mixed with another blander oil e.g. vegetable oil to make salad dressings.

Use to fry tofu (again alone or mixed with another oil) in stir fries and add a dash to Chinese, Thai or Japanese dishes for that authentic flavour.

IT'S YOUR CHOICE...

Unlike many nut and seed oils sesame oil is extremely stable and can keep for years – even in a warm cupboard or worktop – without becoming rancid. Worth bearing in mind next time you go to the shops.

SUNFLOWER

Helianthus annuus L

A valuable source of polyunsaturated fatty acids, both raw seeds and sprouted seeds also contain protein fibre, vitamins B, D, E and K, and a host of minerals and trace plus a wealth of plant chemicals.

Long before Christopher Columbus set foot on American soil, native Americans were cultivating sunflowers not just for food but as a medicine to treat colds, coughs and other respiratory problems. These bright, cheerful members of the daisy family arrived in Europe in 1510, originally as ornamental specimens, but within two centuries they were being widely cultivated for their oil in France and Bavaria, a practice that spread to eastern Europe and Russia, still the world's biggest producer of sunflower oil today.

Although perhaps best known for their oil, sunflower seeds are great as a nutritious snack and one that could have considerable health benefits. In fact, it seems that sunflower seeds and sprouted sunflower seeds are antioxidant, antimicrobial, antidiabetic, help reduce high blood pressure and have wound-healing properties. That's quite a list so let's examine some of them.

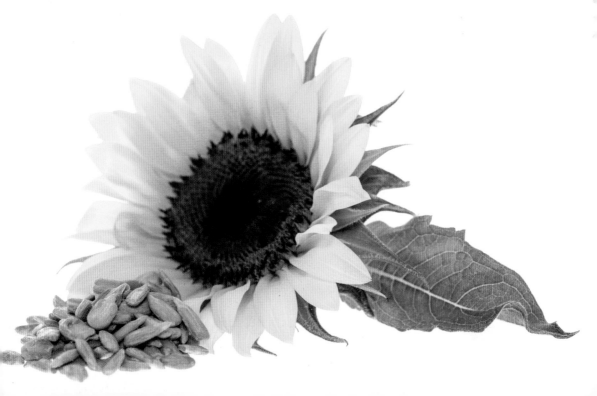

HEART

Sunflower seeds contain several nutrients linked with heart health including vitamin E, the B vitamin, folate, magnesium but most especially those PUFAs and in particular the omega-6 fatty acid, linoleic acid (LA), which according to studies reduces total cholesterol and 'bad' LDL cholesterol, although it also lowers 'good' HDL cholesterol, which is possibly not so desirable.

Indeed, back in the 1960s, it was thanks to this abundant supply of LA that led to sunflower-seed oil becoming the basis for some of the earliest 'nutraceuticals', the fat spreads and oils promoted for heart health back in the day when doctors first linked heart disease to the saturated fats found in animal fats. Remember those tubs of margarine emblazoned with big yellow sunflowers?

CHEWING THE FAT

But the story got muddier over the years, because sunflower oil's high PUFA content meant it was especially susceptible to oxidation so to prevent this – and to make it more spreadable – it was partially hydrogenated. Hydrogenation creates a group of fatty acids called transfats, which are now known to be particularly harmful to the heart and blood vessels. Indeed some experts argue that although LA is an essential fatty acid – meaning that our bodies can't make it so we need to get it from food – in excess it may damage rather than benefit the heart.

All of this led to headlines such as 'Heart attack risks in healthy spreads'. It's a thorny issue that the experts still can't agree upon. But the upshot is that over the past few years, manufacturers have reformulated products to eliminate or significantly lower transfats, although sunflower spreads and oils have not quite reached the dizzy heights of their popularity in the mid-twentieth century.

But science never stays still for long and, as is often the case, the story turns out to be more complicated than the headlines make out. Recently, scientists have identified other compounds in sunflower seeds that could potentially aid heart health, the most promising being plant sterols, which according to research can help reduce cholesterol.

Meanwhile, in an attempt to minimise the downside and harness the potential benefits of LA, food scientists have developed new forms of sunflower oil with a high percentage of oleic acid, the main fatty acid found in olive oil. As you already know if you've got this far, oleic acid is one of the most important heart-friendly nutrients for people consuming a Mediterranean diet, so the thinking is that high-oleic sunflower oil could have benefits for cardiovascular health.

And sure enough, according to a wide-ranging review published in *Advances in Nutrition*, replacing those partially hydrogenated oils with high-oleic oils such as high-oleic sunflower oil could indeed help reduce levels of harmful blood fats and reduce the risk of heart disease. The studies in this review included one which estimated that replacing 7.5 per cent of energy from partially hydrogenated vegetable oils with an equivalent amount of high-oleic sunflower oil could reduce the risk of heart disease by 15.9 per cent. So while there are still questions that remain unanswered, if you like the flavour of sunflower oil or spread, there could be a place for the high oleic variety in the kitchen cupboard.

As for sunflower seeds, fatty acids are not the only potentially heart-protective compounds you could get from a handful. In a study reported in *Food Chemistry* scientists from China identified three 'new' antioxidant nutrients in sunflower seeds. These belong to a family of phytochemicals known as terpenes also found in grape skins – that, at least in a test tube, protected against oxidative damage to heart muscle cells. So it seems there's no need to write off sunflower seeds and their oils just yet.

THYROID

Along with Brazil nuts, sunflower seeds (and sunflower oil), are one of the relatively few non-animal sources of the antioxidant trace element, selenium. This explains why they are regulars on top-ten lists of foods containing selenium, which in small amounts together with iodine is vital for a healthy thyroid, whose job it is to regulate metabolism (our body's ability to break down food and transform it into energy). In fact, as you'll know if you've read the entry on Brazil nuts, of all our organs, the thyroid contains the highest amount of selenium per gram of body tissue, so clearly it's important we get enough of this vital trace mineral.

It's not just our thyroid that requires selenium. Research shows we need it for a healthy immune system, fertility and more (see page 33 Brazil nuts). There's no specific research on sunflower seeds for thyroid disease or to help combat other health problems, so we don't know if they could help, but as part of an overall healthy diet they could be part of that vital synergy between nutrients that helps us stay well.

But a word of caution: remember balance is all and when it comes to selenium, too much can be as damaging to health as too little. You would be hard pushed, to get too much from sunflower seeds unless you really went to town, but snacking on a handful from time to time could help you reach your selenium quota.

CANCER

In Venezuelan traditional medicine sunflower seeds are used in cancer treatment. Although their benefits are purely anecdotal, sunflower seeds do contain lignans, those phytochemicals which have been arousing a lot of interest lately for their potential to help protect against cancer. And one small German study reported in the journal *Nutrition and Cancer* did find that postmenopausal women who consumed sunflower seeds, pumpkin seeds and soybeans, had a lower risk of breast cancer compared with women who had not consumed them.

Of course this could simply reflect that these women were healthy diet savvy. And, you'll know by now to take small studies that haven't been replicated with a fairly hefty pinch of salt. What's more this research was what's called a case control study, meaning that people who have developed a disease are identified and their past exposure to factors such as dietary ingredients is compared with that of other people who do not have the disease. It's one of the least reliable types of evidence, so maybe this is one to watch rather than take as gospel.

DIABETES

Chemicals called advanced glycation end products (AGEs) formed when there are high levels of glucose in the blood contribute to the development of diabetes. Sprouted sunflower seeds may help combat this thanks to the presence of a wealth of potent antioxidant and blood glucose lowering phytochemicals, according to a review published in *Chemistry Central Journal*. One of these chemicals, cynarin, is 8 per cent higher in sunflower sprouts than in another common source artichoke leaves, often used in supplements to help support healthy levels of blood glucose. In rat studies at least sunflower seed extracts help to lower blood glucose as well as improving body weight, the amount of glucose in the liver and many other features of diabetes. Other chemicals in sunflower-seed extract reduce carbohydrate digestion and absorption of blood glucose in the gut. Animal studies are just a start of course but these are interesting findings so keep an eye out for more research.

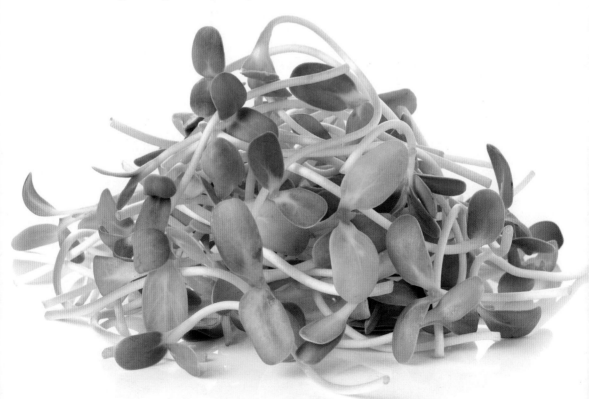

OTHER POTENTIAL BENEFITS

Sunflower seeds contain around 20 per cent of sulphur-rich proteins, a store of essential nutrients the sunflower plant needs to grow and develop after the seed has germinated. According to a review published in the *Chemistry Central Journal* these can help meet several of the body's needs including fuelling muscular and skeletal cell development, insulin production, and acting as an antioxidant. Sunflower oil, at least in rats, helps combat inflammation due to oxidative damage in the stomach, while vitamin E components found in sunflower seeds are also anti-inflammatory. Sunflower oil applied topically to the skin has been found to help wound-healing in animals, while it's suggested that its high-linoleic acid content could even help reverse and cure scaly skin caused by eczema, although the studies are all over the place so it is impossible to draw any clear conclusions or make firm recommendations as yet.

IN THE KITCHEN

Sprinkle toasted, raw or sprouted sunflower seeds with other nuts and seeds on salads.

Add them toasted or raw to muesli, granola or other breakfast cereal for a healthy crunch.

Top bread and cakes with a handful of sunflower seeds before baking.

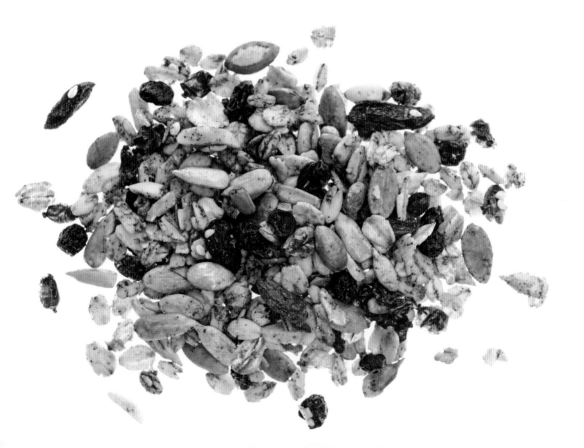

Mix other nuts and seeds such as pumpkin and hazelnuts, dried fruit and rolled porridge oats with sunflower seeds, butter or oil and honey and bake for a tasty, high-nutrient flapjack or breakfast bar.

Combine with bulgur wheat, quinoa, lentils, soya beans and kale for a delicious and nutritious salad.

Add them to scrambled eggs or tofu to add flavour and texture.

Grind them and use to dredge meat and fish instead of flour before frying.

Mix with other seeds, such as sesame or pumpkin; nuts such as cashews and pecans, and dried fruit such as goji berries or dried sour cherries to make a nutritious trail mix.

Swap sunflower seed butter for peanut butter for a change.

Use high oleic sunflower seed oil as a salad dressing.

IT'S YOUR CHOICE...

Sprout sunflower seeds to maximise antioxidant capacity. There are no specific studies looking at how much sprouting increases this in sunflower seeds specifically, but if other seeds are anything to go by, it can be considerable – for example, sprouted mung beans have twelve times the antioxidant capacity of the unsprouted seeds.

WALNUTS

Juglans regia

Finally, to the granddaddy of them all: walnuts. Among the most popular and also well-researched of tree nuts, walnuts, with their startling resemblance to the two halves of a human brain, are one nut, above all, that appear to well-deserve their health-promoting reputation. Studies suggest they may lower the risk of heart disease, type 2 diabetes, reduce symptoms of age-linked conditions affecting the brain and, as part of a healthy diet, help prevent certain cancers.

Walnuts have been part of our diet for at least 9,000 years and cultivated since 4000 BCE by the ancient Greeks, who are thought to have appreciated their health

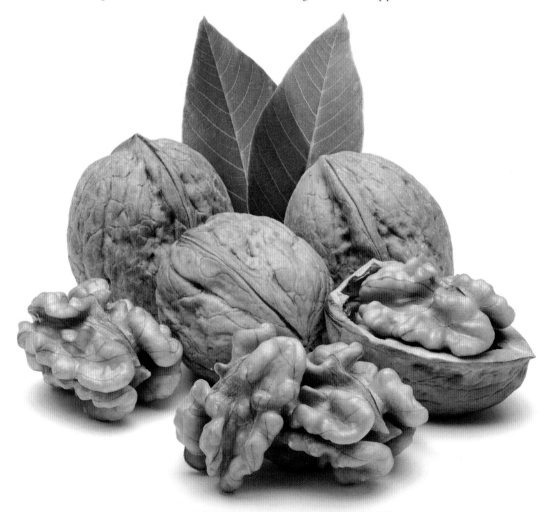

benefits. In the twenty-first century the European Food Safety Authority, EFSA, has allowed the claim: 'Walnuts contribute to the improvement of the elasticity of the blood vessels'. A prized accolade indeed given how hard it is to get official endorsement for such claims and one that is well-deserved.

Of all the tree nuts, walnuts have the best ratio of omega-3 to omega-6 PUFAs – something which some scientists at least believe can benefit both heart and brain health. In particular, one of the fatty acids they contain – the omega-3 plant PUFA, ALA or alpha-linolenic acid – is thought to be partly responsible for protecting the health of participants in the famous Spanish Mediterranean Diet study (PREDIMED).

But it is not just walnuts' fatty-acid content that scientists now think could benefit health. Walnuts abound in other nutrients – think protein, fibre, vitamins B6, folic acid and high levels of the gamma-tocopherol form of vitamin E, plus the minerals copper, manganese and phosphorus.

They also contain the highest known levels of those polyphenols that are attracting so much research attention of any tree nut. Hardly surprising then that they have also been found to have the most potent antioxidant activity of all nuts being second only to rose hips in their antioxidant power. How could all this lead to potential health benefits?

HEART

The ability of walnuts to lower risk factors for heart disease, such as high levels of harmful blood fats, has long been recognised. This explains why they are among the nuts which feature in many of the trials showing that eating nuts in general can benefit the heart. But what about walnuts specifically? World experts from Harvard University examined the results of thirteen trials including 365 people in one of the earliest overviews to examine this question published in the *American Journal of Clinical Nutrition*. They concluded that a diet rich in walnuts helped lower both total and 'bad' HDL cholesterol.

Since the publication of this study in 2009, the understanding of how heart disease develops and progresses has increased. Scientists now have a much more sophisticated understanding of the effects of different types of blood fats on atherosclerosis (hardening and narrowing of the arteries). And in particular heart disease and strokes, are now recognised as being part of a spectrum of so-called cardiometabolic disorders. These start with chemical disturbances such as changes in the way the body processes blood fats and blood glucose. They also include changes in the way the elastic inner-lining of the arteries, the endothelium, behaves. Many of these are driven by oxidation (the human equivalent of rusting) and inflammation.

A randomised controlled clinical trial published in the journal *Metabolism* reflects this new understanding. It involved forty healthy men and women, aged on average

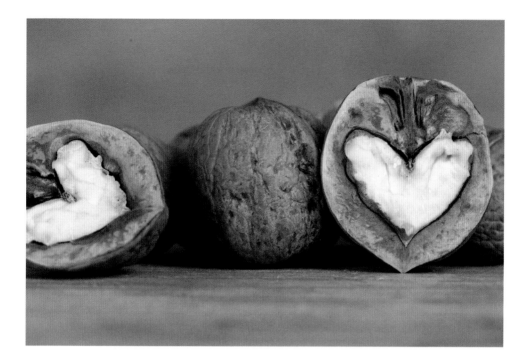

60 years, who first ate a diet with 43 g of added walnuts a day followed by a typical Western diet with no walnuts added or vice versa. Each diet phase lasted eight weeks separated by a two-week-off period. At the end of each diet phase, researchers measured a whole host of markers of inflammation and oxidation. They found that, adding walnuts significantly lowered two key markers of non-HDL cholesterol, a measure that provides a better clue to the risk for heart disease than measuring only LDL, as well as apolipoprotein-B, a component of blood fats involved in atherosclerosis, furring and narrowing of the arteries, and cardiovascular disease. There were no significant changes in the other markers.

This was a small but revealing study which throws light on how regular walnut consumption may lower the risk of heart disease. Yet another study in the journal *Clinical Nutrition*, meanwhile, found that walnut consumption was linked to greater elasticity of the blood vessels. All good news, which strengthens the claims that walnuts have benefits for heart health.

DIABETES AND PRE-DIABETES

Reflecting this new understanding of a spectrum of cardiometabolic disease, researchers have re-examined data from some of the seminal studies which included the effects of nuts on the heart to see what effect they may have on diabetes and pre-diabetes. In one such study, researchers from Harvard University looked at the links between walnut consumption and type 2 diabetes in two large groups of women who took part in two famous studies: the Nurses' Health Study (1998–2008), and the Nurses' Health Study 2 (1999–2009). This involved tracking 58,063 women from the first study, and 79,893 women all free of diabetes at the beginning of studies. It revealed that the more walnuts the women consumed, the lower their risk of developing type 2 diabetes, just one of several studies suggesting that walnuts may help protect against type 2 diabetes.

How might walnuts have this protective effect? Studies suggest that they can improve sensitivity to the hormone insulin and, in doing so, help the body keep blood glucose levels better balanced, something that in turn can slow or halt the development to type 2 diabetes. A recent study in pre-diabetic mice, meanwhile, published in the journal *Nutrients* found that eating the equivalent of a handful of walnuts a day resulted in significant benefits in their ability to use insulin and lowered blood pressure, although it seemed to have harmful effects on blood fats, all of which points to the need for a long-term study in humans.

WEIGHT

One way in which walnuts may benefit cardiometabolic health is by their effects on weight. And this certainly seems borne out by a study published in the *Nutrition Journal*, in which researchers examined the effects of adding walnuts to a low-calorie diet on weight, satiety – feeling full – and risk factors for heart disease. The participants – 100 overweight and obese men and women – were asked to rate their hunger, satiety and how much food they anticipated eating at the next meal at three different time points.

The result? Although both groups lost weight and centimetres around their waist, only those who added walnuts to their diet sustained a drop in systolic blood pressure at six months and also had lower total cholesterol and LDL cholesterol. The study provides evidence that a low-calorie diet that includes walnuts is as effective – and with the added bonus of reducing heart disease risk factors – as a standard low-calorie diet.

In other research published in the journal *Diabetes Obesity and Metabolism* researchers used real-time brain scans to open a window onto the brains of ten people who consumed either a smoothie with added walnuts, or one without walnuts. Guess what? A small area of the brain that helps regulate hunger and appetite was activated in those who drank the walnut smoothie, a finding that suggests that adding walnuts to your diet could help curb cravings if you're watching weight.

BRAIN

If you've got this far you'll be more than familiar with the mantra: 'What is good for the heart is good for the brain', so it's not surprising that evidence is emerging that eating walnuts may benefit brain health too, especially as we get older. The famous

Spanish PREDIMED Study, for example, looking at the benefits of a Mediterranean diet, found that of all nuts, walnuts were the ones most linked to improvements in working memory. This is the type of memory we use in our everyday lives to help us keep shopping lists, phone numbers and other short-term things in mind.

Walnuts certainly have more than a share of potentially brain-friendly nutrients. For a start they're rich in that plant omega-3 PUFA, ALA, which has been found to combat oxidative stress in the brain as well as reducing the death of brain cells, helping them to stay flexible, curbing inflammation, and reducing deposits of the protein 'plaques' found in the brains of people with Alzheimer's disease.

But it isn't all about ALA, according to a paper published in *Frontiers in Aging Neuroscience*. Walnuts also contain the amino acid, arginine, changes in the processing of which are suspected to be involved in the early development of Alzheimer's, plus vitamin E, folate and a wealth of those polyphenols that help keep blood pressure stable, increase levels of 'good' HDL cholesterol and help maintain the elasticity of the arteries.

How might all these play out? In a review published in the *Journal of Nutrition*, researchers from the highly regarded Human Nutrition Research Center on Aging at America's Tufts University, suggests that walnuts, walnut oil, and the nutrients they contain may help protect memory and preserve brain function as we get older. This could in turn help to fend off cognitive decline and dementia. The researchers conclude that, 'Taken together, this evidence suggests that the integration of walnuts into a healthy diet could be an effective means of prolonging health spans, slowing the processes of brain aging, and reducing the risk of chronic neurodegenerative disease.'

And it's not just dementia that walnuts might help protect against. According to a study in *Neurochemical Research*, they also appear able to reverse the degeneration of brain cells in Parkinson's disease – in mice at any rate. Other studies, meanwhile, hint that they may help banish depression and improve mood.

The trouble is that, despite all these studies, there's not yet anything firm or conclusive enough on which to base a clear health message. Enter the Walnuts and Healthy Aging Study (WAHA), a clinical trial set up to explore the role of walnuts in maintaining the health of the brain and the retina, which lies at the back of our eyes.

During the study, which ran from 2012 to 2014, 708 men and women aged 60 years on average followed their normal everyday diet with half adding around 30 to 60 grams of walnuts a day. Full results are awaited but findings from a 'sub-study' reveal that regular walnut consumption lowers high blood pressure in older people with a low risk of heart disease. A message worth taking on board. I for one am really looking forward to further results.

CANCER

The research is nowhere near as advanced as it is for the heart and brain. Nevertheless, as the authors of a review in the *Journal of Nutrition and Cancer* suggest, those omega-3

PUFAs, vitamin E, plant sterols and plant chemical in walnuts could also have the power to help protect against cancer.

Indeed, animal studies in which walnuts were added to the diet have found that walnuts block the rate of growth of breast cancer cells and slow the growth of prostate, colon, and kidney cancers. How? It seems they help staunch the formation of blood vessels that fuel these cancers and stop cancer cells from proliferating. Fascinating findings that, if translated into humans, suggest yet another good reason for adding walnuts to our diet.

GUT

How might walnuts exert their potentially cancer preventive effects? As so often, it could come down to their effects on the gut. A study published in the *Journal of Nutrition*, for example, looked at the effects of walnuts on gut bacteria. In this study, of eighteen healthy men and women from the Washington area aged between 25 and 75 years, eating walnuts boosted levels of three types of beneficial gut bacteria. Eating walnuts also the lowered the percentage of two chemicals linked with an increased risk of bowel cancer. It seems we don't absorb all the calories in walnuts – meaning that the undigested residue acts as a 'prebiotic', or fertiliser, for gut bacteria to get to work on. Yet another shout-out for the benefits of walnuts.

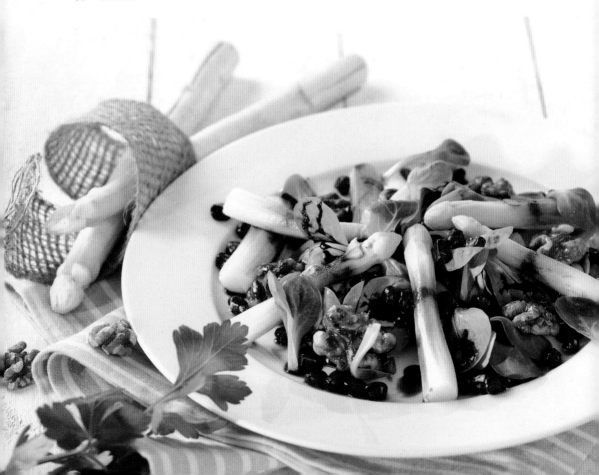

IN THE KITCHEN

Add whole or halved to other nuts for a healthy snack.

Chop and sprinkle over salads, porridge, muesli and other cereals.

Roast or toast and add to homemade granola.

Add a handful to your morning smoothie mix to help you stay full and satisfied until lunchtime.

Dry fry until crisp in a little oil then sprinkle over sweet and savoury dishes such as lentil soup.

Add to stews and casseroles – cooked walnuts are essential in many Persian dishes such as the sweet-sour stew *fesenjan*.

Pounded or ground with parsley, walnuts to make a great alternative to basil and pinenut pesto. Spoon over spaghetti or spiralised courgettes (courgetti) or add to tahini sauce.

Add a few walnuts and grapes to a cheese board – they go especially well with blue cheeses such as Roquefort.

Swap olive oil for walnut oil in salad dressings or drizzle over pasta, fish or poultry.

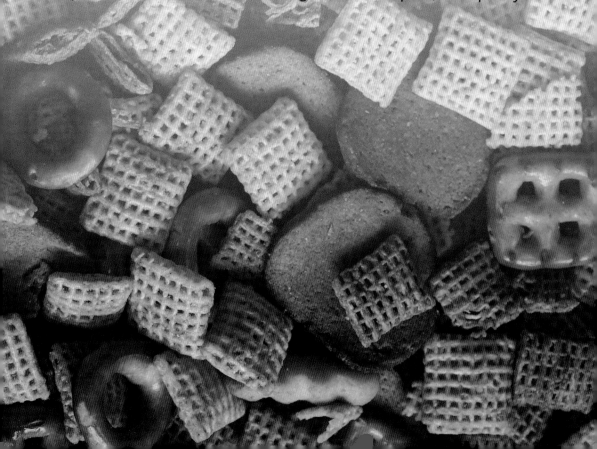

THE NUTS AND BOLTS

I f there's one message I hope you've gained from this book it's that individual foods and nutrients are less important than the synergy between them as part of a healthy diet. So, while the nutrients below, are some of the most important found in nuts and seeds, the best way to get their benefits is to eat a good variety of different ones as part of an overall healthy dietary pattern.

ALPHA-LINOLENIC ACID (ALA)

One of two essential fatty acids we have to get from food, as our body can't make them (see also Linoleic Acid). A plant form of omega-3, ALA gets longer in the body to form two other omega-3s found in oily fish, which the body finds easier to use. Contemporary Western diets are relatively short of omega-3s compared to omega-6s, which some think may contribute to chronic diseases such as heart disease and dementia. Chia seeds, flaxseeds and walnuts and their oils all contain ALA, which it is thought may help account for some of their benefits for the heart and brain.

AMINO ACIDS (AAS)

The 'building blocks' of protein responsible for many processes in the body. They include nine 'essential' AAs we have to get from food as we can't make them in our body. Among many reasons are advanced for the potentially beneficial effects of nuts on the arteries, their low content of the amino acid, lysine, compared to their relatively high content of another amino acid, arginine is thought to be one of the most important. Arginine changes into nitric oxide in the body, which helps keep blood vessels elastic and improves blood flow.

ANTIOXIDANTS

Natural compounds that help to prevent oxidation, a process akin to rusting, which happens when oxygen reacts with other chemicals. Oxidation is thought to be partly responsible for damaging the genetic material or DNA inside our cells, which is in turn linked to many chronic diseases. The classic antioxidants are the so-called ACE vitamins C, E and beta-carotene, which is converted into vitamin A in the body, plus the trace element, selenium. Many of the health benefits of nuts and seeds are thought to be due to the antioxidant properties of both these and other nutrients including phytochemicals.

BUTYRATE

A so-called short-chain fatty acid (SCFA) synthesised by gut bacteria from undigested carbohydrates including fibre. Researchers now think that butyrate and other compounds produced when gut bacteria get to work on fibre is responsible for the benefits of high fibre foods such as nuts and seeds (as well as fruit, veg, pulses and wholegrains). Butyrate is important for gut health and some research suggests it may have a role in helping to prevent colon cancer. It may also have beneficial effects for several conditions including high cholesterol, insulin resistance and ischaemic strokes, the type when a blood clot or other blockage cuts off the blood supply to the brain.

CARBOHYDRATES

One of the big three macronutrients that are converted to glucose in our body and used by our cells as a source of energy for our organs and muscles. Nuts and seeds are relatively low in carbohydrates and the ones they do contain are unrefined carbohydrates as opposed to the refined variety found in cakes, pastries, sweets and biscuits.

FATTY ACIDS

The form in which fats come in food. There are several types – saturated, monounsaturated and polyunsaturated fatty acids (SFAs, MUFAs and PUFAs). These can also be classified as short chain, medium chain and long chain. Most foods including nuts and seeds contain a mixture of different fatty acids.

FIBRE

Plant-based carbohydrates that pass unabsorbed or undigested through our small intestine – where we absorb most nutrients from food – to the large intestine or colon where our gut bacteria get to work on them. They include plant components such as lignans, found in plant cell walls. Insoluble fibre – what we used to know as roughage – in nuts increases satiety or feelings of fullness and bulks out our stools. Soluble fibre absorbs water turning into a gluey, gel-like substance that feeds gut bacteria. It slows digestion of other nutrients helping prevent blood glucose spikes and increases production of bile acid, which carries cholesterol out of the body. These classifications of fibre are changing. Experts are still arguing over exactly how to get this message across, but one thing is certain: according to the World Health Organisation and national nutritional advisory bodies we need around 30 grams a day for health, and nuts are definitely a part of how we can reach this.

LINOLEIC ACID (LA)

The other 'essential fatty' acid. LA is an omega-6 PUFA. LA also gets longer in the body to form another fatty acid called arachidonic acid (AA), which provides structural support to cell membranes. It's important for enabling cells to communicate with each other and coordinate their actions (cell signalling). We need both omega-6 and omega-3 fatty acids. Some experts believe, however, that our Western diet contains too many omega-6s relative to omega-3's and that this is partly responsible for many chronic diseases.

MACRONUTRIENTS

Nutrients our bodies need in large quantities. There are three: carbohydrates, fats and protein.

MICRONUTRIENTS

Nutrients our bodies need in small quantities. They include all the vitamins and minerals and so-called trace elements like selenium that we need in minute quantities.

MINERALS

Micronutrients found naturally in soil and water and absorbed by plants. We get them from eating their leaves, fruit, stems or seeds or the meat of animals which have fed on them. Minerals are needed for a host of bodily functions – for example calcium for strong bones and heart, iron for healthy red blood cells, potassium for regulating blood pressure. Different nuts and seeds provide varying amounts of different minerals. For example Brazil nuts are rich in selenium, almonds in calcium, cashew nuts in iron and pistachios in potassium. Another good reason to mix things up.

MONOUNSATURATED FATTY ACIDS (MUFAS)

A type of fatty acid that is liquid at room temperature. The most abundant MUFA in nuts and some seeds is oleic acid, the main fatty acid in olive oil, which is thought to be partly responsible for the heart-healthy properties of the Mediterranean diet. MUFAs unlike PUFAs are highly resistant to oxidation, which could in part explain their effects.

PHYTONUTRIENTS

Plant chemicals produced by plants to protect them against predators and disease. With a wide range of biological actions in the body, another name for them is bioactives. Some phytochemicals are pigments, which give plants their colour, hence the advice to 'Eat a rainbow'. Some protect against UV light. others provide flavour and scent either to attract animals that can help them spread or pollinate their seeds, or to repel pests. Many hundreds have been identified to date and there are still more being discovered. One of the biggest classes of phytochemicals are polyphenols widely found in nuts and seeds.

PHYTOSTEROLS

Plant chemicals with a similar chemical structure to cholesterol that have been shown to lower blood levels of cholesterol. Phytosterols 'compete' with cholesterol from the diet in the liver, where most of the cholesterol in our body is made. This increases the amount of cholesterol excreted, and decreases the absorption of cholesterol in the intestine. Sesame seeds have the highest amount of phytosterols and Brazil nuts the lowest. Pistachio nuts and sunflower seeds are the nuts and seeds richest in phytosterols.

POLYPHENOLS

A large class of phytochemicals found in nuts and seeds often in their skins. Antioxidant and anti-inflammatory they also work in a host of other ways to keep cells healthy. Polyphenols are thought to be responsible for many of the benefits of nuts such as lowering blood pressure and increasing the elasticity of arteries. Raw and roasted walnuts have the highest polyphenol concentration of any nuts. Polyphenols work in synergy with other nutrients. For example, almond polyphenols work with alpha-tocopherol (see Vitamins) to block oxidation of LDL cholesterol, a key stage in the development of atherosclerosis, furring and narrowing of the arteries.

POLYUNSATURATED FATTY ACIDS (PUFAS)

Liquid at room temperature, the two main types are: omega-3s and omega-6s. They are important parts of cell membranes needed to make many substances in the body and helping cells work properly. Omega-3s are thought to decrease inflammation, while a surfeit of omega-6s is thought to increase it. Omega-3s have been found to be important for heart and brain health. Omega-3s and omega-6s battle it out for the same chemical 'pathways' in the body and some experts think the relative ratio influences the risk of disease, although the optimal ratio has never been definitively identified. PUFAs in nuts and seeds are thought to be partly responsible for the lower risk of heart and associated diseases in regular nut eaters. PUFAs, however, are highly susceptible to oxidation which is what makes nuts and seeds and their oils so prone to rancidity – and a reason why you need to store them properly and use quickly.

PREBIOTICS

Food components, such as fibre, that escape digestion in the small intestine or upper bowel and stimulate fermentation in the bowel increasing the amount of healthy gut bacteria and producing secondary chemicals which have other potential health effects. This is increasingly thought to be one of the key reasons accounting for the health benefits of nuts.

PROBIOTICS

One of the biggest buzz words in nutritional science at the moment, probiotics – aka friendly, good or healthy bacteria – is the term used for the bacteria and other micro-organisms that live in the large intestine or colon. They have a wide range of effects on gut health and the immune system. The effects of nuts and seeds on helping to promote these good gut bacteria are thought to be a key reason for their health benefits.

PROTEIN

One of the three macronutrients needed to build and repair tissues. Containing between 9 and 20 per cent, nuts and seeds, despite their small size, are relatively rich in protein

SATURATED FATTY ACIDS (SFAS)

Usually solid at room temperature, SFAs are most often more abundant in foods of animal origin. They have been linked to higher levels of total and 'bad' LDL cholesterol. However, nutritional scientists are reaching a greater understanding of saturated fats and have found that some are less harmful than others and some may even be beneficial. Let's just say 'it's complicated'! Nuts and seeds contain small amounts of some SFAs which work in synergy with the other fatty acids they contain.

VITAMINS

Chemicals made by plants and animals which we eat and our bodies need to function. There are thirteen: vitamins A, C, D, E, K and the B vitamins (thiamine, riboflavin, pantothenic acid, biotin, vitamin B6, vitamin B12 and folate). In an ideal world get all the vitamins we need from our food and we also make vitamin D in our skin, and vitamin K in our gut. Of particular relevance to nuts is the antioxidant, vitamin E, which comes in several different forms called tocopherols and tocotrienols. Although alpha-tocopherol is the most common form, gamma-tocopherol which is abundant in nuts is thought to work in harmony with alpha-tocopherol to protect cells from oxidative damage.

THE HIERARCHY OF EVIDENCE

Who can you believe when it comes to nutrition - someone you met at a party, a post on social media, a health professional or published research? When nutrition experts weigh up the evidence they look to published research. But different kinds of studies have different strengths and shortcomings. Enter the hierarchy of evidence which ranks research in terms of reliability.

THE PROS AND CONS

The hierarchy of evidence is not a perfect system when it comes to food and nutrition. However, despite its drawbacks, when many different types of studies all point the same way it's a fair cop.

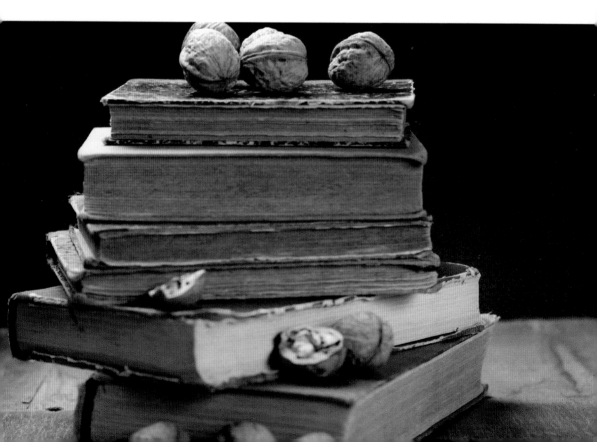

A hierarchy-of-evidence pyramid with three columns: **Type of study**, **What it is**, and **Pros and cons**.

Type of study	What it is	Pros and cons
Systematic review/ meta-analysis	Overview of studies which collects together evidence from lots of other studies to reach a conclusion	Considered top of the tree as it provides the strongest, most robust evidence though to an extent it depends on the quality of the original studies included.
Randomised controlled clinical trial (RCT)	Two or more groups of people are randomly allocated to receive a particular food/diet/nutrient. One group receives the food/diet/nutrient under scrutiny. The other (control) group receives an alternative, placebo or dummy treatment.	Well-designed RCTs can be great but they can be expensive and often last too short a time to give meaningful answers. The more people in an RCT the more reliable the findings. A big drawback in nutritional RCTs is the difficulty of creating a placebo as it's not easy to disguise what someone is eating!
Observational study	These include several types of study e.g. cohort studies in which a group of similar people (a cohort) is followed over a long period to see whether a particular food/diet/nutrient affects a particular outcome such as heart disease, diabetes or the risk of dying.	These sorts of studies come in for a lot of flack – mainly because although they can show associations or links between a food /diet/ nutrient and a health outcome they can't prove cause and effect. However they can give strong clues as to the effects of different diets/foods/nutrients that can then be investigated in other studies.
Lab-based studies	Test tube and animal studies carried out in the lab. These can give clues to how a particular nutrient/food/diet may affect cells or animals.	Can throw light on mechanisms but bear in mind cells in a petrie dish are different to whole bodies. And rats and mice aren't humans! Findings may not carry over into people so view with a degree of caution.
Expert opinion	As the name suggests this is the view of a qualified expert/doctor/professional body.	Has the weight of informed experience behind it but still an opinion and as such considered a relatively weak level of evidence.
Anecdote	This can be anything from traditional usage to what you heard on the grapevine or read on Instagram, Twitter and the rest.	Interesting – sometimes - but unreliable evidence and at the worst 'fake news' nonetheless!

SELECTED REFERENCES

Alasalvar C, Bolling B.W., Review of nut phytochemicals, fat-soluble bioactives, antioxidant components and health effects. Br J Nutr. 2015 Apr;113 Suppl 2:S68-78.

Assaf-Balut C, García de la Torre N, Durán A, Fuentes M et al. A Mediterranean diet with additional extra virgin olive oil and pistachios reduces the incidence of gestational diabetes mellitus (GDM): A randomised controlled trial: The St. Carlos GDM prevention study. PLoS One. 2017 Oct 19;12(10):e0185873.

Aune D, Keum N, Giovannucci E, Fadnes L.T., Boffetta P, Greenwood DC, Tonstad S, Vatten L.J., Riboli E, Norat, Nut consumption and risk of cardiovascular disease, total cancer, all-cause and cause-specific mortality: a systematic review and dose-response meta-analysis of prospective studies. BMC Med. 2016 Dec 5;14(1):207.

Bitok E, Sabaté J, Nuts and Cardiovascular Disease. Prog Cardiovasc Dis. 2018 May 22. pii: S0033-0620(18)30092-6.

Bolling B.W., Chen C.Y., McKay D.L., Blumberg J.B., Tree nut phytochemicals: composition, antioxidant capacity, bioactivity, impact factors. A systematic review of almonds, Brazils, cashews, hazelnuts, macadamias, pecans, pine nuts, pistachios and walnuts. Nutr Res Rev. 2011 Dec;24(2):244-75.

Casas-Agustench P, Salas-Huetos A, Salas-Salvadó J, Mediterranean nuts: origins, ancient medicinal benefits and symbolism. Public Health Nutr. 2011 Dec;14(12A):2296-301.

Cunningham E. What are n-7 fatty acids and are there health benefits associated with them? J Acad Nutr Diet. 2015 Feb;115(2):324

Chon S.U., Total polyphenols and bioactivity of seeds and sprouts in several legumes. Curr Pharm Des. 2013;19(34):6112-24.

de Souza R.G.M., Schincaglia R.M., Pimentel G.D., Mota J.F., Nuts and Human Health Outcomes: A Systematic Review. Nutrients. 2017 Dec 2;9(12).

Falasca M., Casari I., Maffucci T, Cancer chemoprevention with nuts. J Natl Cancer Inst. 2014 Sep 10;106(9)

Flores-Mateo G, Rojas-Rueda D, Basora J, Ros E, Salas-Salvadó J, Nut intake and adiposity: meta-analysis of clinical trials. Am J Clin Nutr. 2013 Jun;97(6):1346-55.

Gorji N, Moeini R, Memariani Z, Almond, hazelnut and walnut, three nuts for neuroprotection in Alzheimer's disease: A neuropharmacological review of their bioactive constituents. Pharmacol Res. 2017 Dec 5.

Guasch-Ferré M, Liu X, Malik V.S., Sun Q, Willett W.C., Manson J.E., Rexrode KM, Li Y., Hu FB, Bhupathiraju SN. Nut Consumption and Risk of Cardiovascular Disease. J Am Coll Cardiol. 2017 Nov 14;70(20):2519-2532

Hayes D, Angove M.J., Tucci J, Dennis C, Walnuts (Juglans regia) Chemical Composition and Research in Human Health. Crit Rev Food Sci Nutr. 2016 Jun 10;56(8):1231-41.

Jackson C.L., Hu F.B., Long-term associations of nut consumption with body weight and obesity. Am J Clin Nutr. 2014 Jul;100 Suppl 1:408S-11S.

Kornsteiner-Krenn M, Wagner K.H., Elmadfa I. Phytosterol content and fatty acid pattern of ten different nut types. Int J Vitam Nutr Res. 2013;83(5):263-70.

Larsson S.C., Drca N, Björck M, Bäck M, Wolk A. Nut consumption and incidence of seven cardiovascular diseases. Heart. 2018 Apr 16.

Papanastasopoulos P, Stebbing J, Nuts and cancer: where are we now? Lancet Oncol. 2013 Nov;14(12):1161-2.

Rajaram S, Valls-Pedret C, Cofán M et al., The Walnuts and Healthy Aging Study (WAHA): Protocol for a Nutritional Intervention Trial with Walnuts on Brain Aging. Front Aging Neurosci. 2017 Jan 10;8:333.

Reynolds A, Mann J, Cummings J, Winter N, Mete E, Te Morenga L. Carbohydrate quality and human health: a series of systematic reviews and meta-analyses. Lancet. 2019 Feb 2;393(10170):434-445.

Ros E, Health benefits of nut consumption. Nutrients. 2010 Jul;2(7):652-82. doi: 10.3390/nu2070683. Epub 2010 Jun 24.

Ros E, Martínez-González MA, Estruch R, Salas-Salvadó J, Fitó M, Martínez JA, Corella D. Mediterranean diet and cardiovascular health: Teachings of the PREDIMED study. Adv Nutr. 2014 May 14;5(3):330S-6S.

Rusu M.E., Gheldiu AM, Mocan A, Vlase L, Popa DS. Anti-aging potential of tree nuts with a focus on the phytochemical composition, molecular mechanisms and thermal stability of major bioactive compounds. Food Funct. 2018 May 23;9(5):2554-2575.

Sabaté J, Ang Y. Nuts and health outcomes: new epidemiologic evidence. Am J Clin Nutr. 2009 May;89(5):1643S-1648S.

Sala-Vila A, Guasch-Ferré M, Hu FB, Sánchez-Tainta A et al; PREDIMED Investigators, B. Dietary α-Linolenic Acid, Marine ω-3 Fatty Acids, and Mortality in a Population With High Fish Consumption: Findings From the PREvención con DIeta MEDiterránea (PREDIMED) Study. J Am Heart Assoc. 2016 Jan 26;5(1).

Valls-Pedret C, Lamuela-Raventós R.M., Medina-Remón A, Quintana M, Corella D, Pintó X, Martínez-González M.Á., Estruch R, Ros E. Polyphenol-rich foods in the Mediterranean diet are associated with better cognitive function in elderly subjects at high cardiovascular risk. J Alzheimers Dis. 2012;29(4):773-82.

van den Brandt P.A., Nieuwenhuis L, Tree nut, peanut, and peanut butter intake and risk of postmenopausal breast cancer: The Netherlands Cohort Study. Cancer Causes Control. 2018 Jan;29(1):63-75.

Xiao Y, Huang W, Peng C, Zhang J, Wong C, Kim J.H., Yeoh E.K., Su X. Effect of nut consumption on vascular endothelial function: A systematic review and meta-analysis of randomised controlled trials. Clin Nutr. 2018 Jun;37(3):831-839.

ABOUT THE AUTHOR

Patsy Westcott is an award-winning freelance journalist, health writer and self-confessed foodie who has written thousands of articles on health and nutrition for national newspapers, magazines and websites. She is as passionate about how what we eat can benefit our health as she is about the science behind it. So much so that she decided to study for a Master of Science degree in Nutritional Medicine at the University of Surrey and graduated in 2014 with distinction.

Patsy has also written or co-authored more than forty popular health books, including *Healthy Eating to Reduce the Risk of Dementia* (Kyle Books), the first evidence-based cookbook designed to help people eat and prepare foods linked with a lower risk of dementia.

A runner up in the British Medical Association Health Awards, 2015, the book, co-authored with Professor Margaret Rayman and dietitians Vanessa Ridland and Katie Sharpe, was commended as 'one of a kind ... [which] presents in a very effective way, useful background information and a full explanation of all the nutrients that help the brain to function as its best for longer.'

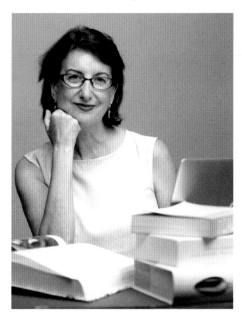

Index

breads 24, 28, 39, 43, 46, 49-50, 65-66, 78, 91, 95, 100-1, 106

breast cancer 14, 17, 27, 33, 48-49, 71, 89, 94, 100, 104, 109, 118

C

calcium 16, 24, 26, 35, 39, 41-42, 57, 63, 80, 85, 100-2, 122

calories 11, 24-25, 37, 70, 85-86, 88, 118

cancer 9, 14, 17, 22, 27, 30, 33, 37, 48-51, 53-54, 70-71, 77, 82-83, 89, 91, 94, 99-101, 104, 109, 113, 117-18, 121

carbohydrates 11, 15, 21, 24, 30, 36, 51, 63, 93, 100, 102, 121-22

cardiovascular 12-14, 25, 30, 36, 40, 53, 68, 70, 76, 85, 99, 103, 108, 115

carotenoids 51

cashews 11, 17, 20, 35-38, 112, 122

catechins 75, 85

cells 10, 15, 21-22, 26-27, 30, 32, 38, 52-53 59-60, 67, 72, 77, 80, 82, 94, 104, 111, 120-24, 126

cereals 39, 83, 91, 101, 119

cerebral atrophy 53

chia seeds 20, 39-43, 90, 120

cholecystokinin (CCK) 81

cholesterol 13, 17, 25-26, 30-33, 35-37, 40, 45-46, 52-53, 58-59, 63, 65, 67, 75-76, 82, 85-86, 93, 97-100, 103, 108, 114-17, 121, 123-24

  HDL 25, 30-31, 37, 40, 52, 58, 63, 75, 85, 98-99, 103, 108, 114-15, 117

  LDL 25-26, 31-32, 36-37, 40, 45-46, 52-53, 63, 65, 75-76, 82, 85-86, 93, 97, 99-100, 103, 108, 115-16, 123-24

coeliac disease (CD) 43, 99-100

cognition 14, 53

colitis 28

colon 11, 17, 27, 54, 104, 118, 121, 124

  cancer 27, 54, 121

constipation 47, 60

copper 16, 26, 30, 69, 80

coronary heart disease (CHD) 68

D

daidzein 99

deaths 9, 14, 53, 68

dementia 10, 22, 26, 53, 99, 117, 120

depression 32, 71-72, 117

diabetes 9, 14, 17, 23-25, 36, 40, 42, 45-47, 63-64, 69-71, 75-76, 82, 84-89, 91, 93, 97-98, 103-4, 110, 113, 115-16, 126

diarrhoea 28, 82

diet 7-8, 12-15, 22-25, 27, 32, 36-37, 40, 42, 46-51, 53-54, 58-59, 61, 63-65, 69, 74-77, 80, 86-88, 90, 94, 97-100, 103-4, 108-10, 113-18, 120, 122-23, 126

digestion 18-19, 21, 43-44, 50, 99, 101, 110, 121, 124

diseases 9-12, 15, 17, 22, 24, 27, 36, 53, 59, 81, 94, 96, 101, 104, 110, 122-23

  bowel 28, 47

  chronic 15, 60, 64, 80, 117, 120, 122

  coeliac 43, 99

  degenerative 17

  neurodegenerative 10

  peripheral arterial 14, 45

  respiratory 9

DNA 15, 30, 32, 52-53, 120

E

eczema 59

eggs 50, 55, 64, 112

energy 24, 39, 41, 48, 67, 104-5, 109, 121

evening primrose 59

eyes 27, 32, 50, 64, 82, 85, 94, 110

F

faeces 31, 46

fats 11, 13-15, 24-26, 29-32, 35-36, 40-42, 45-47, 51-52, 54, 57-59, 63-64, 68-69, 74-76, 79-82, 85-88, 91, 94, 97-99, 102-4, 108, 114-16, 121-22, 124

fatty acids 15, 19, 23-24, 26, 37, 39, 54, 57, 59, 63-64, 67, 74-75, 80, 82, 89-91, 98-99, 103, 107-9, 114, 120-24